Against All Odds

Against All Odds

The Life of Kishore V. Sonpal

HETAL SONPAL

RUPA

Published by
Rupa Publications India Pvt. Ltd 2021
7/16, Ansari Road, Daryaganj
New Delhi 110002

Sales centres:
Allahabad Bengaluru Chennai
Hyderabad Jaipur Kathmandu
Kolkata Mumbai

ISBN: 978-93-91256-11-1

First impression 2021

10 9 8 7 6 5 4 3 2 1

Printed at Parksons Graphics Pvt. Ltd, Mumbai

CONTENTS

FOREWORD

Usually, only the lives of great men are recorded; only in exceptional cases are the lives of certain ordinary people also recorded and captured in the form of a book. These books tell stories of the extraordinary way in which they lived their life and impacted the lives of many others. Their life lessons become valuable and educate future generations. Shri Sonpal was one such person.

I was very pleased when Shri Sonpal's son, Hetal, approached me to write the foreword to Shri Sonpal's biography. The story of a man like Shri Sonpal should be known and shared for others to learn from. Through this book, Hetal has brought Shri Sonpal back to life. *Against All Odds* describes intricate details about the challenges Shri Sonpal faced in his childhood, funding his own engineering and then shares the story of his fifty-year-long professional career, where he served various organisations with integrity, valour and a great deal of hard work. He was a man of integrity and total devotion, and the various instances in his life shared in this biography, further describe how he did not compromise on his principles, despite all the hardships he had to face.

I got to know Shri Sonpal a little more than a decade ago

when he joined the Bharatiya Vidya Bhavan as the Registrar of the Coimbatore Kendra. To begin with, our relationship was quite formal. However, as we got to know each other better, our relationship became closer and went beyond the limits of the Bhavan. I grew fond of him and soon, he was more a friend than just my colleague.

Retirement, for many, is a nightmare. That was not the case for Shri Sonpal. His religious bent of mind and his training in yoga and meditation helped him move away from a hectic professional career to the calm and serene atmosphere in the Bhavan.

Times are getting challenging, and time-tested values of our world are all slowly but surely disappearing. The need for leaders with a high sense of integrity and morality will only continue to grow and the absence of good men like Shri Sonpal will be felt deeply. If at all there is a dearth of anything today, it is that we no longer find men of character and commitment. Many great institutions, otherwise blessed with everything—like resources, infrastructure and goodwill—realise that it is difficult to find leaders who can work with them for greater glory. Shri Sonpal belonged to a generation that had seen, observed and even worked with great men, and had imbibed their qualities. We hope for the tribe to grow if India has to advance in keeping with the country's potential.

I got to know Hetal more intimately only after the passing of his father, Shri Sonpal. In many ways, Hetal has inherited most of the noble qualities of his father. His relationship with Shri Sonpal was more than that of a father and a son; it was more like that of a teacher and a disciple. This relationship, so rare in today's material mundane world, is quite evident in many instances within the biography.

Shri Sonpal was a well-read man with great admiration for spiritual masters and political leaders. Reading was his passion and he has left behind a huge collection of books. It is befitting for a man of Shri Sonpal's stature to have his own biography. This book will be a great source of inspiration for many youngsters who can learn from his life and figure out how to handle their own challenges.

I wish Hetal the very best in his new journey as an author.

Dr B.K. KRISHNARAJ VANAVARAYAR,
Chairman,
Bharatiya Vidya Bhavan,
Coimbatore

PREFACE

Sometime in June 2019, Lata called her son, Hetal in Gurgaon and informed him that Kishore's appetite had reduced. His father had become frail, lacked energy and slept for fourteen/ fifteen hours every day. Hetal immediately suggested that Lata get a blood test done for Kishore.

The test report showed that his platelet count was low, so the doctor suggested further tests. Subsequent tests confirmed what was feared. *Kishore had late-stage prostate cancer.* Hetal received the report over an email, and tried in vain to decipher the technical terms below the high-resolution images of his father's body. Hetal then spoke to the family physician about the report, who suggested palliative treatment. The term was new to Hetal and his jaw dropped when the search results were displayed on the computer, *Care for the terminally ill.* Hetal was dumbstruck and muttered, *'No, I won't let cancer take my Pappa away'.*

Hetal immediately booked a flight to Coimbatore, and flew out the next day. An appointment was fixed with an oncologist. The doctor reviewed Kishore's reports and suggested hormone therapy as the first stage of treatment. Cancer thrives on hormones in the body and the injection would stop the body from producing any more of them.

While they were all waiting for the injection to be administered, Hetal said something that lit up Kishore's face and brought a sparkle in his eyes. He said, 'You have to help me write your biography.'

The next day, Kishore was on the phone, calling people and telling them, 'My son is writing a book about me!'

1

THE BIG FALL

Only those who dare to fail greatly can ever achieve greatly.

—Robert F. Kennedy

It was a chilly and windy morning in February of 1938. Vinodrai was inspecting the kitchen as workers and cooks were going around, supervising last-minute preparations as the big day was approaching.

Two months back, after a tough bidding war, his company, Surti Sweet Mart, had won its biggest contract, an order to make whopping 8,000 kilograms of sweets for one of the biggest annual events in the country, the Congress Adhiveshan (Assembly Session). The Indian National Congress, with more than seventy thousand members, was the largest political party in the country and the convention was to be their grandest event.

The location of the event was to be Haripura, a small town

approximately seventy kilometres away from the industrious and bustling city of Surat. The brief to Vinodrai was to serve the delegates of the Congress something that they would find in a traditional Gujarati village. The session was to be the first of the newly appointed leader, Subhash Chandra Bose and had gained prominence as a number of crucial decisions were to be taken during the meeting.

It was Sardar Vallabh Bhai Patel who had chosen Haripura as the venue for the convention. Fifty-one bullock chariots had been decorated. Nandalal Bose, one of the pioneers of modern Indian art, had created a set of seven posters at the request of Mahatma Gandhi, while film director, J.B.H. Wadia of Wadia Moviestan Studio, had filmed a feature-length documentary for the occasion. This event was a big deal for a middle-level businessman like Vinodrai.

Vinodrai's father, Ramji Madhavji, was a prosperous sweet merchant. Originally from Amreli, Ramji Bhai, along with his three brothers, had established sweet shops in Surat, before settling in Ahmedabad and setting up three sweet shops there. They lived in one of the famous suburbs of Ahmedabad, known as Paldi.

Vinodrai was married to Mangala Ben, who also hailed from a prominent family in Ahmedabad. Mangala Ben's father was a self-made man and owned a fruits business and resided in a palatial bungalow in Ahmedabad. In the early 1900s, he had started off as a simple road-side vegetable seller. Gradually, through sheer hard work, he expanded into wholesale fruit business.

Vinodrai had not left any stone unturned in preparing for the Adhiveshan; procuring the best ingredients (flour, dry fruits, sugar, etc.) and hiring the best cooks. Vinodrai even took a loan to execute the project as he refused to take a single paisa in advance for the event owing to his nationalistic feelings.

With just a day to go, all the preparations were complete and the ingredients and utensils were kept ready in a pandal at the venue. Unfortunately, the weather Gods played truant. What looked like ominous dark clouds threatening light showers, turned out to be a massive cyclone. The lashing rain washed away the entire kitchen, including ingredients and utensils. Vinodrai and his men tried in vain to salvage whatever they could.

Without any insurance to cover such a disaster, the burden of the huge loss hit Vinodrai immensely. He was left with no choice but to sell off his house, office and all his possessions to repay his creditors. What could have been his greatest achievement ended up becoming his biggest disaster. Now, penniless and helpless, the family hoped for a new beginning. On 21 August 1938, on the cusp of a new life, Vinodrai's wife, Mangala Ben, gave birth to their first child, Kishore.

2

THE FORMATIVE YEARS

Growing old is unavoidable, but never growing up is possible. I believe you can retain certain things from your childhood if you protect them—certain traits, certain places where you don't let the world go.

—Martin Luther King, Jr.

Kishore Thakkar grew up in Ahmedabad, the largest city in the western state of now Gujarat. Born soon after the family had gone through a huge financial setback, Kishore had a tough childhood. Shuttling between Ahmedabad and Bombay (as Mumbai was then called), Kishore's childhood was quite eventful and full of challenges. Call it fate or God's will; Kishore was being prepared for the tougher times ahead.

In summer of 1942, his paternal grandfather, Ramji Bhai, moved from Ahmedabad to Bombay, and took up a job with the Police. Soon after in the month of August, Mahatma Gandhi started the Quit India Movement, encouraging the freedom fighters to free India from the clutches of the British. Congress and the Socialist leaders expected to capture seats of power in major cities by the first week of August; they wanted to control the villages and rural areas by the second week. However, things did not go as per plan. By 18th August, the revolution that was to culminate in the capture of power collapsed and the whole nation was forced to deal with the counter-measures of British repression. Lakhs of people were arrested throughout India; in Bombay alone, 1,028 people were killed, 3,214 were wounded and more than 10,000 people were jailed.

Ramji Bhai, being part of the Bombay Police, was disturbed at having to arrest his own people. He hailed from a family that practiced principles of non-violence as propagated by Mahatma Gandhi. Therefore, Ramji Bhai decided to quit the police job.

Ramji Bhai was a businessman at heart, but to initially build up some savings, he worked at various sweet shops till he finally settled in, working with his uncle, Jayanti Bhai, at the famous sweet shop in South Bombay, Amarchand Sukhadia.

His grandparents adored Kishore. When he was just five-year-old, Kishore's parents took him, along with his younger brother Jagadish, to the Ahmedabad Railway Station to meet his grandparents, who were on their way back to Bombay after a pilgrimage to the holy city of Dwarka.

At the station, after exchanging pleasantries and handing over the Prasad to his parents, his grandmother (Dadima) asked Kishore, 'Kishore, why don't you come and stay with us in Bombay? We will get you admitted in the local school and you can live next to the beach.' Even before his parents could answer, Kishore answered, 'YES.'

Kishore quickly bid farewell to his sobbing mother (also called 'Ba'), father (fondly called 'Bhai') and Jagadish before boarding the train. Being poor, all that Kishore had were two sets of clothes but Dadima assured they would get new ones in Bombay.

Kishore was fortunate enough to be welcomed by a large family at his grandparents' house in Bombay. His uncle, Jayanti Bhai, aunt Bhabhu and Faiba (father's sister) all lived together in a small house in South Bombay. His grandfather and his uncle together worked hard to provide them a simple life. They got Kishore admitted into Grade 2 in the local municipal school.

Their house was opposite the Dunlop tyre factory, next to the famous Yak Tailor, five hundred meters from the famous Chowpatty Beach. Kishore enjoyed time at the beach and quickly fell in love with the city. He often missed his parents, and when he was in Grade 3, his grandparents noticed his homesickness and felt that he should return to his parents. At the end of that school year, Kishore returned to his hometown and joined a local school in Girdhar Nagar in Ahmedabad.

At the time of registration in the local municipal school, his new surname, Sonpal, was formalized. Henceforth, he would be known as Kishore Sonpal. It was a challenge for Vinodrai to place his eldest son in a private school with the meager salary he earned as a clerk in a local mill. Out of his monthly salary of fourteen rupees, he had to account for the house rent of six rupees and monthly expenses of seven rupees with a monthly saving of one rupee. Vinodrai had to work in multiple shifts to make ends meet. Although Mangala Ben was from a well-to-do-family, Vinodrai refused to ask for help. He was content with his simple clerical job and his respectable salary. Their house had six occupants with just one water tap for shower and other requirements. Mangala Ben, being the only lady, would shower in the house, while all others had to shower in the open. Mangala Ben's wardrobe consisted of just two sarees. Even buying a Bindi was considered an avoidable purchase.

Kishore's parents did not have an easy life and were struggling to make ends meet. Mangala Ben, in just those three years, had given birth to three children (two girls and one boy), but none of them survived. After the two boys, Mangala Ben was keen to have a daughter and had her first girl child; she was adorable. When she was a few months old, the child developed a small tumor on the back of her head. It seemed insignificant initially, but grew bigger within a week. As they could not afford the two rupees needed for checkup by a regular doctor, Mangala Ben went to the local vaid (doctor). Mangala Ben applied the balm given by the vaid on the child's head, but it had no effect and after a few hours, the child died. The family was shocked and saddened by this tragedy. The subsequent child had to be aborted to save Mangala Ben's life.

Subsequently, Mangala Ben gave birth to their third child and first daughter, Jyoti. Jyoti had chicken pox soon after her birth and was ill for a long time. Once she recovered, the long fight with the disease left her very weak. She started walking only when she was five. She had to be carried around everywhere till then. Their fourth and youngest child, Renuka was born two years after Jyoti. The family was thus complete.

As a nine-year-old, Kishore walked five kilometres every day to school as the school bus was beyond their means. But Kishore made good use of this opportunity to discover shortcuts to the school, traipsing through residential areas and farmland. By the time he reached Grade 5, he had had his share of fun. He would leave school early sometimes, on the pretext of a holiday or an inspection and have fun playing with the neighbourhood kids.

After a few months of settling down, at around the time of Diwali, Kishore was out playing with other kids and accidentally stepped on a piece of glass. It pierced through his foot and hurt terribly. He took out the glass shard and limped back home in great pain. Mangala Ben applied some tincture and wrapped it with a cloth. But walking barefoot worsened the wound and it grew infected. After almost a month of suffering like this, Vinodrai was able to arrange funds to buy Kishore a pair of chappals. The whole incident made Kishore realise the perils of poverty and the kind of compromise they had to make, even for proper medical support.

Kishore was introduced to the concept of fasting early in his childhood by Vinodrai; he would keep different fasts on days like Saatam, Aatham and Ekadashi, nine days of Navratri, month-long fast in the month of Shravan and even a four-month-long fast where he ate only one meal a day. In hindsight, fasting was a good way to address the challenge of poverty; rarely were two sumptuous meals in the day guaranteed anyway.

Kishore also learned early to never borrow from anyone or take loans. One day, he was only eight when there was a knock on the door. His father had gone out, only his mother was at home with the kids. A man had come to deliver a summons from the court. Kishore's father had defaulted on the repayment of a loan he had taken from his colleague in the mill. Kishore's mother was aghast on hearing this.

When his father came home a great argument ensued, and Kishore got to know the whole story. Vinodrai was a simple worker earning a meagre salary. When Mangala Ben was six months pregnant Vinodrai was worried about the expenses for the upcoming delivery. Leave alone money for hospital, it was tough to afford a horse-cart ride to the hospital. It was this quandary that made him take the extreme step of borrowing money. When it came to repayment he did not have the funds. He had not imagined his colleague would go to court for something this trivial.

Not wanting the issue to haunt them, Mangala Ben somehow secured whatever cash needed to repay the loan. Observing the pains that his parents endured due to the loan, Kishore decided never to borrow money from anyone.

As an immediate consequence of the financial setback, the family adopted new set of measures to save money. They further cut down on the small list of permissible vegetables; quantity of oil to be used for cooking was reduced as well. His father was able to get a six-month waiver on Kishore's school fees. After six months, he was moved to the municipality school farther away from home. Kishore's commute time increased, but it was worth it, as this school did not charge any fees.

Being poor did not prevent his family from being kind. His mother believed in feeding others before feeding her children. The first chapatti was always saved for the cow, and the second one was for the neighbourhood dog. Even on days when food was not cooked, Kishore was told to buy grass to feed the cows near the Babul Nath temple near their house. These small acts of kindness and generosity laid the foundation in Kishore's mind about the virtues of sharing.

Another time, some of his friends suggested that they watch a movie together. A new Raj Kapoor movie was released and he was Kishore's favourite actor. However, Kishore hesitated as he had school the next day. Kishore was a quiet child. While his friends were naughty, loved cracking jokes and playing pranks, Kishore remained serious and focused on his studies. His humble background made Kishore determined to study hard. He wanted to get a good job and give his family a better life. He did not like the idea of missing school. What will he tell his teacher?

'Oh, that's easy, you just tell your teacher that you are sick,' his friends suggested. Kishore rarely missed school, even when he was genuinely not well. So he thought for long in the bed at night, debating on lying to his teacher or missing the movie and finally decided to seek the advice of the school Principal.

'Sir, I would not like to lie that I am not well and go for the movie,' Kishore said explaining to his principal the next day. 'But if I tell the truth, then I am denied the chance to enjoy a movie with my friends. What should I do?' The principal was a strict disciplinarian, but he understood the young child's quandary. He told Kishore that as long as his lie was not causing anyone harm, as an exception, it was acceptable that he went to watch the film. Kishore was relieved and happily went with his friends.

A few months later, Kishore faced yet another challenge that taught him integrity. Kishore and Jagadish used to commute together by bus at the time. Due to his short height, Jagadish would get away by purchasing only a half-ticket. Thus, they would save money to buy a small packet of dry gram, *or* chana, a great treat. On one such occasion, their mother noticed a yellow stain on Jagadish's shirt pocket and enquired about it.

'Oh, we had some chana the other day,' exclaimed Jagadish. His father looked at Kishore in surprise and inquired about the money for the chana. He was flabbergasted when he heard about the half ticket and made them promise never to cheat the bus conductor (and God) ever again. Kishore vowed not to do something like this again.

In another instance, he learnt a lesson about gambling. His uncle was fond of gambling, and had made a lot of money from it; he would often let Kishore and the other kids play various card games, including the famous Indian card game, *Teen Patti* with one rupee each. But an incident narrated one day by his father, made Kishore decide never to gamble in his life.

It was evening and Vinodrai was ambling back home, tired to the bone. As he crossed the marketplace, he heard the loud cries of a vendor.

'Come, come and challenge your luck with the roll of a dice! Double your money! come, come take a chance, try your luck!'

Vinodrai's feet dragged. The groceries were pending, house rent was overdue and medicines had to be bought. But his hand was thoughtfully kneading the lone five-rupee note in his pocket. The vendor was cajoling. 'Come on Babuji, try your luck once.' Vinodrai gave in. He placed a bet with his sole five-rupee note, closed his eyes and rolled the dice.

He won.

'Your money has doubled now! Fortune braves the player. Here is your money, Babuji!' the vendor loudly exclaimed. Vinodrai was elated. His eyes gleamed.

'Babuji, what is the point of just one try, today is your lucky day. Take the dice and roll it on your lucky number,' the vendor persisted.

Vinodrai tried again. He chose his lucky number and pledged ten rupees, and won again. His happiness knew no bounds as he felt the twenty rupees in his hand. His mind was racing. Another two rounds would ease all his worries. He imagined the joy when he would take the handsome amount home. Just *two* more chances.

With the newfound confidence, Vinodrai rolled the dice on his favourite number. The dice rolled and tossed, hitting his favourite number, it took a final turn and fell flat.

He had lost.

He clenched his fists. With the twenty rupees, he had lost his hard-earned five rupees too. He felt ashamed. He did not want to go home with an empty pocket. Yet he had lost, he had no choice and no money to reclaim any of his lost money and pride. He turned around to leave.

'O Babuji,' called the vendor, 'it is just one game you have lost. Do not worry. Fortune favours the brave, remember?'

'I have no more money,' he replied.

'Don't worry about money,' the vendor said to his surprise. 'Who is asking for money to try your luck? You can pledge your ring and get earnings in cash,' the vendor gleefully coaxed.

Vinodrai considered it. The vendor pulled him close. 'Try your luck with this ring on your lucky number.'

The ring was worth about hundred rupees. Two hundred would be a princely amount for Vinodrai if he won. Reluctance and desperation tugged his heart. The vendor kept encouraging him to play. With a heavy heart he pulled his ring out and pledged. His trembling hands shook and rolled the dice one last time on his lucky number.

Unfortunately, Vinodrai lost.

He walked away despondent. He was not sure how he would share what had happened with his wife. When he reached home and described his shame, Mangala Ben was very upset. She could not believe that Vinodrai would do such a thing. She scolded him. She had been working hard, saving small amounts every month from his meagre salary, and this kind of loss made a huge dent in their savings. She contacted Mohanlal Masa, Kishore's uncle. He had connections in the neighbourhood where the roadside gambler operated. Mohanlal Masa immediately went to the vendor and was able to get Vinodrai's ring back from him.

Incidentally, later Mohanlal Masa himself lost all his wealth, including his house and car in gambling. It was irony that the messiah who helped Vinodrai recuperate his gambled loss, himself ended up penniless due to the vice. After the unfortunate incident of the ring and what happened with Mohanlal Masa, Kishore was clear that he would never gamble in his life.

This was the time when India's fight for independence was coming to an end. Kishore was deeply influenced by the leaders of that time. Mahatma Gandhi, Jawaharlal Nehru and Acharya Vinoba Bhave were his role models. At 11 p.m. on 14 August 1947, their father took Kishore and Jagadish on his cycle to witness the celebrations. India had finally gained independence from the British Raj. While the essence of this Independence was not clear to the kids, they did not mind the pomp, the nice music and the sweets they got to eat.

Kishore often loved going to his maternal grandfather's house. When Nanaji (maternal grandfather) died early in his sixties, his mama (maternal uncle) would take care of Kishore. Being the eldest child, he had to represent the family at social gatherings. He would attend many grand weddings and receive his fair share of delicious sweets.

His paternal grandfather, Ramji Bhai was close to his extended family. Every year, he would make a few trips to meet all the relatives in native places of Virpur, Amreli, Rajkot and elsewhere. On many of these trips, he would take Kishore and Jagadish along. From a young age, Kishore grew close to many of his relatives. This helped him to establish bonds with all his relatives and he became very popular. These were foundational traits of networking learned by Kishore—to not only meet a lot of people, but also remember them and stay connected.

In summer of 1948, the kids travelled to Bombay with their grandmother for the janoi (a thread ceremony among the Hindus) of his uncle, Arvind kaka. His grandmother again doted on him and when she heard about the poor quality of education in the municipal school in Ahmedabad, she suggested that the kids should resume schooling in Bombay. Vinodrai agreed, and both the kids were admitted into the Nutan Kelavani Mandir School in South Bombay.

Kishore was now getting familiar with Bombay. He enjoyed himself thoroughly there, riding on horse carriages, visiting the fast-food stalls that served delightful snacks and *kulfi* (Indian ice cream) by the beach. The tram ride to the famous Taj Mahal Hotel, Apollo Bunder, then sitting on small rides there were activities that excited Kishore and he used to look forward to these. Of course, these were expensive outings reserved for special occasions.

While his uncle, Jayanti Bhai, worked at a local sweet shop, Amarchand Sukhadia in the Zaveri Bazaar area of Bombay, his wife, Bhabu, used to manage the house. To increase the earnings, Bhabhu would make badam puri (almond cake) from fresh almonds. It became extremely popular in the locality and was also sold to the sweet shops for a premium.

Kishore and Jagadish were roped in to not only make the

puri, but also to go to Chowpatty and sell the badam puri in the evening after school. They would start from Mafatlal Bath near Chowpatty, and cover the entire 3-kilometre stretch on foot to Nariman Point, shouting, '*Badam Puri le lo, Badam Puri!*' (Almond cake, please buy some almond cake) Normally, they would make two rupees in the day. On a lucky day, they might collect five rupees.

At the end of the day, when they looked forward to a comfortable night's sleep, it was not always granted. With not enough space in the house for all, when they had guests over, Kishore and Jagadish along with their uncle, would even sleep on the footpath.

At the time, Kishore's grandfather's former partner from his sweet business encouraged him to join him in the new business in Vile Parle. He was even able to get Kishore's uncle, Jayanti Bhai and father Vinodrai to join. And slowly, the Sonpal family settled in Bombay.

It was in Nutan School in Bombay that Kishore made some of his closest friends. Pravin Dalal, Gajendra Shah and Krishnakumar Merchant were in the same class as Kishore. Pravin, coming from a wealthy family, was always lion-hearted. Kishore looked forward to going to his palatial house in Walkeshawar. Together they played kho-kho and other sports at the beach, and helped themselves to some occasional snacks. Other close friends from school were Surya Kumar Soda and Niti Tanna. Their roll numbers were close to Kishore's, thus began a strong friendship that would last decades. Niti, was the aunt of Lata Parmanand Popat, whom Kishore would marry many years later.

Having studied in a Gujarati-medium in Ahmedabad and in English-medium in Bombay, Kishore did not have an easy time in school. It was through his will power and strong memory that Kishore was able to excel. Kishore was behind by a year in English, and it took him time to catch up with the others.

They often visited the landmark Eros theatre in Bombay and it was here he watched his first English movie. Pravin had bought the tickets for *Chase a Crooked Shadow.* Watching movies was another way for Kishore to improve his English. However, in mathematics, Kishore and Pravin were both wizards and could solve the toughest problems with relative ease.

Whenever he had the chance, Kishore would rush to listen to the great personalities speak at events. He was greatly influenced by Acharya Vinoba Bhave. Before he heard him, Kishore believed that Vinoba Bhave was a lady, as his first name ended with the suffix 'ba'. His friends could not stop laughing when the truth was revealed when they all heard Vinoba Bhave speak at a rally. Kishore was all of twelve at that time, but he remembered the speech by Acharyaji and became his lifelong bhakt (devotee).

After he passed the seventh grade, he joined the National High School in Ahmedabad. He would remain there till his matriculation. He missed his friends in Bombay, and looked forward to meeting them during summer vacations.

While Kishore was in Ahmedabad, Vinodrai was in Bombay for work in the city. Being the eldest, Kishore was now the head of the family. He took care of everyone, helping Mangala Ben with household chores as well as taking care of his younger siblings. Even at that young age, he had perfected the art of sleeping early and rising at Brahma Muhurta.

Although he was a strict elder brother, he had a good sense of humour as well. During the Paush Purnima Vrat (a ritual practised by sisters to pray for the long and healthy life of their brothers), the sisters would sing the song:

Poshi Poshi Poonamdi, aakhashe randhi kheer,
Vrat kere che ben ane jame chey veer.
Bhai ne ben jame ke rame?

(Lovely full-moon night, the sky has cooked a sweet porridge;
Sister is fasting and brother is having a delicious dinner:
Sisters are asking: should we play or eat?)

In the last line of the song was a question addressed to the brother; the sisters would ask—should we play or eat dinner? Kishore would tease his sisters, and announce that he would play all night. But he would later smile, and lovingly ask them to break their fast.

Despite being in separate cities, Pravin and Kishore's friendship grew deeper over the years and it was Pravin who encouraged Kishore to consider joining the famous Wilson College in Bombay after high school. However, Kishore could not make the cut-off points needed for Wilson and instead opted for Jai Hind College in Bombay. He would study science there for the next four years.

3

FIRST ENGINEER IN THE FAMILY

If people knew how hard I worked to achieve my mastery, it wouldn't seem so wonderful after all.

—Michelangelo

June 1957. Kishore was studying Inter-science at Jai Hind College in Bombay and India was plagued by one of the worst epidemics. The virus was first identified in February 1957, it was then considered as among the 'least severe' of the three influenza pandemics of the 20th century. But it followed the Spanish flu in severity. Between May 1957 and February 1958 more than four million cases were reported in India, with thousand plus deaths in a population of 360 million (according to the 1951 Census). Around the world, about two million people died.

Back then, medical facilities available in India were very basic. Doctors did not have the tools to diagnose diseases or antibiotics to fight secondary infections. *In those days, hospitals were places you went to die, not to get treated.*

Among the millions impacted, nineteen-year-old Kishore too was a victim. He was living in his parents' house in Kandivali; a simple cough soon transformed into a 104-degree fever. He was shifted to his uncle's house at Chowpatty. Despite the medical treatment his uncle procured for him, Kishore's situation did not improve. By the twelfth day, his fever rose further by two degrees. The thermometers back then were not even calibrated to measure higher temperatures. Kishore slipped in and out of consciousness and would frequently talk gibberish. His uncle and aunt, fearing the worst, called his parents over from Kandivali.

The house was not large enough to accommodate them all, so Kishore and his parents shifted to a relative's house in Vile Parle. Better medical facilities were available in the suburbs and the doctor there immediately suggested a blood test. The test results confirmed that he had typhoid. He was immediately administered treatment. Typically, the virus of typhoid prevails for 7-10 days, but he had been sick for all of 21 days. As he had developed ulcers in his mouth and stomach, his diet was restricted to moong dal (green gram) water and fresh limejuice. By the end of April, he had been sick for almost a month.

As May rolled in, his health was improving. But it was only by the second week of June that Kishore could resume college. He started commuting by train from his home in Vile Parle to Jai Hind College in South Bombay.

Once he resumed college, Kishore focused on his studies, catching up on what he had missed. His upcoming final exams would decide which engineering college he would join. He frequently walked the streets near Nariman Point, observing roadside vendors, especially those selling books or stamps. He would observe the display of stamps from different countries, covering a wide range of topics. For Kishore, who had a limited view of the world outside of Mumbai and Ahmedabad, the stamps, packed in sets of fifty or hundred, neatly placed on cardboard and protected from dust with polythene, were literally a window to the world. While he had no money to buy the stamps then, he was confident that he would have his own stamp collection one day.

In 1957, career options were grossly limited, and Kishore was considering colleges in Delhi and Roorkee. During weekends, he discussed with Pravin and deliberated on the high fees and the need for a domicile certificate for applying to colleges in other states. All of this worried Kishore greatly.

However, all the preparations came to naught when the Inter Science final results were declared. Kishore had secured only 57 per cent in the final and would not get admission in any engineering college. He would have to do a three-year diploma course. And so, he moved to Government Polytechnic (RCT) in Ahmedabad. Once again, he bid farewell to the city of Bombay, his family and friends.

While he was not aware of it at the time, Kishore would go on to make a new set of close friends including Shailesh Mehta, Gajendra Shah and Sardar Variyam Singh. In fact, Kishore, Shailesh and Variyam Singh were so often seen together in RCT, that they were popularly known as 'The Three Musketeers'. The days spent in RCT were memorable ones for Kishore. Apart from long lectures, which he attended with lot of seriousness, he enjoyed the time spent in the canteen with his friends, cracking jokes, talking about the future of the country and where their careers would take them.

Though Kishore had accepted the reality of the diploma course he had not given up his dream to become an engineer. He was determined to make the most of another opportunity, whenever it came. Back in those days, students who secured first class in the third and final year of their diploma had an option to join in the second year of engineering.

Kishore worked very hard and secured a seat to study electrical engineering in LD College in Ahmedabad. However, Variyam Singh and Shailesh were not as lucky, and they took up jobs in the city. Back in Bombay, call it irony or fate, Pravin had had a setback. The very friend who encouraged Kishore to be an engineer had to give up his own engineering dreams. Pravin's father, Shri Dwarkadas Dalal, suddenly passed away and he was entrusted the task of handling the family business. Pravin did continue his studies, and chose to pursue law locally from the National Law College in Bombay.

By now Kishore's parents had settled in Bombay permanently. His sisters, Jyoti and Renuka, were also in Bombay. Kishore rushed to Bombay to share the good news about LD with his family. When he entered the house Mangala Ben was busy preparing dinner in the kitchen and Vinodrai had just reached home from work.

'Bhai, I have some good news. I got my diploma results and I have secured admission in LD College for engineering!' Kishore shared his news with lot of excitement. They were elated, but a tinge of sorrow snaked in. Vinodrai did not have funds to pay for the course; Kishore would have to fund his engineering course by himself.

LD Engineering College was one of the oldest and most prestigious colleges of Gujarat, about 15 kilometres away from Kishore's home in Girdhar Nagar. As he was going to stay alone, Kishore had to figure his life out. His First Class in Diploma also got him a scholarship, which reduced the fees burden partially. To pay the rest, Kishore found a job at a coaching centre, where his task was to set questions and correct test papers. He soon settled into a routine. Kishore had the house to himself and did not have a complicated routine. His morning routine included boiling a bowl of green gram for breakfast. After breakfast, Kishore would run to catch the bus. He would have lunch at the canteen—a simple vada or some snacks. In the evening, he would leave from college by 5:30 p.m. and take a bus to reach the coaching centre by 7 p.m. He left the centre at 8:30 p.m. and would prefer walking after that. He would pick up a packet of peanuts or roasted chickpeas to eat while walking back home. This would invariably be his dinner for the day.

As the years passed, his hard work paid off. Kishore became the first engineer in the Sonpal family. His determined effort inspired Jagadish, Jyoti and Renuka also to pursue higher education and set career goals. Not to be satisfied with graduation, he encouraged them to pursue a Master's degree as well. This made everyone, including RamjiBhai—his grandfather, very happy and proud of Kishore's ability to motivate others in the family.

4

ONBOARD THE RAILWAYS

I am looking for a lot of men who have an infinite capacity to know what cannot be done.

—Henry Ford

After graduating as an electrical engineer in 1964, Kishore applied for a job in the Indian Railways. In order to keep his options open, he also applied for the position of senior engineer at Bhabha Atomic Research Centre (BARC) and to teach as assistant lecturer in his own college. But he had a gut feeling that he would make it into the Railways. As a fresh engineer, he preferred a job that could challenge him to continue learning, one he would enjoy doing. However, he also had to take into account his family and consider the compensation. While congratulating him on becoming an engineer, his father had told him clearly, 'Kishore, now you need to take charge of the house and take care of Ba. I cannot manage it anymore.' He would have to keep his promise.

BARC called him in for a written test and interview. Fortunately or not, Kishore did not clear it. Soon after, he received a call from the Indian Railways.

He cleared the tests and on his birthday, 21 August 1964, received his offer letter from the Southern Railways. He had been appointed as an Electrical Engineer. His first posting was to be in Hubli, Karnataka. He had hoped for posting in Madras (now Chennai), the headquarters for the Southern Railways. At that time, Kishore didn't even know about the existence of a city named Hubli.

While Kishore was contemplating the long journey ahead, he reached out to a relative travelling a little further from Hubli, a place called Karwar. He agreed to accompany Kishore till Hubli. The relative also gave him a reference—he was to get in touch with Amrutlal Singada of Saurashtra Automobiles. Mr Singada was a known personality in Hubli and was familiar with the city.

Upon reaching Hubli, Mr Singada helped Kishore find accommodation at a lodge. The lodge had its own rules, which included the payment of a monthly rent in advance. At the time Kishore had only twenty-five rupees, much below the stipulated amount, and requested the lodge owner to allow him time until his first salary was cleared to pay the rent. This is how his life began in Hubli.

His workplace, the railway workshop was only three kilometres away from the lodge; an easy walking distance for someone used to travelling longer distances in school days. Kishore would leave at 8 a.m., drop in for lunch at the lodge and return back tired at 5 in the evening. His meals were remarkably simple—a cup of tea or coffee in the morning, a rice plate at lunch, a banana as an evening snack and some biscuits and tea for dinner.

The salary was paid on the 25th of every month, but as

Kishore joined a few days later, he missed out the first month's salary. He waited out the month of September, and finally received his first salary. He received 425 rupees, a princely amount for young Kishore, who had never seen so much money in his life. It was a momentous occasion and he went to the nearby temple to thank God.

Kishore was fortunate to meet Mr Vaidyanathan, a foreman with the Railways, early on in his career. They grew to become fast friends. Mr Vaidyanathan and his wife resided in a spacious three-bedroom apartment and they invited Kishore to move in and occupy one of the spare bedrooms. Kishore graciously accepted the offer and moved in during the second month. The Vaidyanathans were warm and hospitable, and Kishore enjoyed the meals that he fondly shared with them. Mrs. Vaidyanathan was very kind, and for a very long time, Kishore would recall the awesome coffee she used to prepare every morning.

At work, Kishore underwent an arduous training session for the first six months. In the first three months he studied the lighting system in the train. His manager, the district engineer, was happy with his work and his contributions.

During one of the sessions, Kishore noticed that a culture of excessive spending was prevalent in the Railways. People would replace parts whenever they would encounter a problem; little thought was given to repairing these faulty products. The dynamo, a major component of the train, was fitted with precious metals like copper and brass. Kishore noted there were about 125 faulty dynamos with the unit, that no one was doing anything about. Kishore decided to take up the issue and contacted the supplier, J Stone & Company (a UK based company with office in Madras) and explained the issue. He let them know that since only the coil and the brushes were damaged these could be replaced and the dynamos could work as they did earlier. The supplier agreed to make the replacement for a small cost.

The unit head and his colleagues were very impressed with Kishore and his unique solution. He had brought down the incurred costs significantly. Thus, Kishore's ingenuity and smart observation saved them over 4,800 rupees for each dynamo. The entire set of 125 dynamos were repaired in a span of three months and put back into service. The senior management of the division was extremely impressed by Kishore's proactiveness in this project and the fact that he went beyond his regular call of duty. In one of the division functions held subsequently, he was given a certificate as a special recognition—he had undertaken a project that ensured that the Railways made a phenomenal savings of more than six lacs rupees annually, for which Kishore was given a princely sum of twenty-five rupees as cash award.

At that time, steam engines were employed in the trains and water was a key component. During his training, Kishore was to understand how water is filled, and overall function and use of the pump. Kishore underwent training at a pump station in Madras for three months. Since the Railways had not provided accommodation, he decided to stay with his cousin, Charu, during that period. His other cousin, Kokila, was also married into the same family and it was a large household. Kishore was lucky to have a room for himself.

Every morning, Kishore left at 6 to head to Perambur for the workshop, via the central Madras railway station. Kishore's work at Perambur was quite hectic. After a long day, he would return at 6.30 in the evening. He was fortunate to have a loving sister, who packed meals for him every morning. Kishore would look forward to dinner with Charu and her family.

While Kishore was posted in Madras, a major dispute erupted over the issue of language. In early 1960s, the state of Madras simmered against the Centre. The central government had named Hindi as the official and national language, which was seen as a forced imposition on non-Hindi speakers. In

1965, when Hindi finally became the official language of India (in accordance with Article 313 of the Indian Constitution), the state of Madras turned into a theatre of protests. The protestors, mostly students, demanded that Chapter 17 of the Indian Constitution, which dealt with the question of the nation's official language, be immediately removed.

When C.N. Annadurai, a brilliant rhetorician both in Tamil and English, argued against the imposition of Hindi during the parliamentary debate on the Official Language Bill in 1965, Bhupesh Gupta of the Communist Party of India (CPI) defended the use of Hindi as the sole official language of multilingual India. During the 1966 language agitation in Madras, the CPI suggested a three-language formula for Tamil speakers—a formula that made Hindi compulsory.

Earlier, when the union government was attempting to make Hindi the official language of India, the Madras Congress collaborated with them by suppressing voices of protest against Hindi.

The 1965 language agitation continued for fifty-five long days. For Kishore, who grew up mostly in Bombay, where Marathi was the prominent language and Hindi was spoken quite frequently and was well accepted, this kind of agitation against Hindi made little sense.

The Madras Congress collaborated with the union government by suppressing voices of protest against Hindi. The Congress government, headed by M. Bhaktavatsalam, let loose a reign of terror. On 10 February 1965, policemen shot dead thirty-five agitators. The brutality did not end even after two ministers from Madras—C. Subramaniam and O.V. Alagesan—resigned from the union cabinet in protest. The notorious Defense of India Act, 1962, enacted in the wake of the Indo-China War, was invoked against these agitators. Finally, state jurisdiction prevailed, and the use of Tamil was allowed for most of the governmental proceedings.

Hailing from North India, Kishore was an outsider in Tamil Nadu. He was considered to be 'pro Hindi', so he was cautioned on possibly being targeted by the agitators if seen around the protests. Thus, Kishore had to plan his commute carefully during the days of the agitation.

Back in Hubli, Kishore's next area of focus was on overhauling of electric coaches. As the Electrical Engineer, Kishore's job was critical to ensure the smooth running of the vehicle. Apart from the engine, Kishore took a proactive interest in other components like the dynamo and pump. This type of positive attitude earned him lot of appreciation in the unit. He was also made responsible for the incentive scheme for engineers at the Hubli unit.

Due to some unforeseen issues, Kishore had to shift out from Mr Vaidyanathan's house after a few months. However, he was lucky to be invited to stay at another senior colleague's house—Mr Patra, who was originally from West Bengal. He had a warm and memorable engagement with Mr Patra.

Over time, the bachelor Kishore built a social circle that ensured that he had a life outside of work. He often met Amrutlal Singada, and also became friends with his son, Ramesh Singada. Kishore would go to meet them at their shop, Saurashtra Automobiles that dealt in automotive parts. They had interesting discussions with many others there, including their close friends, Mr Bhailal and Mr Nattu. A wide range of topics, including spirituality, religion and politics, were discussed. Kishore expanded his knowledge and got a better perspective of life through these discussions.

In the meanwhile, the country was going through a crisis with tension on the border. The Indo-Pakistan War of 1965 was a culmination of skirmishes that took place between the two countries from April to September 1965. The conflict began following Pakistan's Operation Gibraltar, which was designed to infiltrate forces into Jammu and Kashmir to precipitate an insurgency against the Indian State. India retaliated by launching a full-scale military attack on West Pakistan. The seventeen-day war caused thousands of casualties on both sides and witnessed the largest engagement of armoured vehicles and the largest tank battle since World War II. Hostilities between the two countries ended after a United Nations-mandated ceasefire was declared, following diplomatic intervention by the Soviet Union and the United States, and the subsequent issuance of the Tashkent Declaration.

Later in month of October, once peace had been restored at the border, Kishore decided to spend the first Diwali of his professional life with his parents in Bombay. While in Bombay, he visited his father's shop and helped in the business, since Diwali was the peak season for sweet shops. Vinodrai was happy to have Kishore helping him during that busy period.

◆

Kishore spent three exciting years, from 1964 to 1967, in Hubli, after which he was due for a promotion. A new, eighth division had been formed by the Indian Railways, known as the South-Central Railway. The Chief Electrical Engineer was promoted and posted in Secunderabad and was keen to have Kishore move with him. Even the District Electrical Engineer supported this decision and ensured that Kishore could make the move to Secunderabad. Kishore was now responsible for the purchasing of all electrical equipment as the new Head of the Department.

Kishore was fortunate to get such a big jump early on in his career. The new role provided him with a large, three-bedroom house in Secunderabad. Kishore set up and furnished his new house in Secunderabad with a lot of interest. The hardships he faced in Hubli were now a thing of the past. Kishore worked extremely hard at his new job. He was soon familiar with all the purchasing activities in the division. He scrutinized and negotiated many crucial tenders, learnt about a larger variety of material to be procured and travelled across the country. He visited all the major cities including Bombay, Madras, Calcutta (now Kolkata), Lucknow and Delhi. Kishore was entitled to a pass that allowed free first-class travel, and on the long tours he often interacted with many senior personnel and managers in different departments. His honest and sincere work was commended, and Kishore found recognition across ranks.

He also accompanied the Chief Electrical Engineer for regular inspections of various units. He was awed by the amenities in the railway coach. There was a steno and first-class cooking facilities for the engineers in this special coach, also known as the A-Class Saloon. The saloon had a drawing hall, a dining hall, kitchen and two separate bedrooms.

During this transition, Kishore made friends with Mr Narasimhan, who was also transferred to Secunderabad. In Hubli, Narasimhan was a stenographer for the DE (District Engineer). When the DE was transferred, he took Narasimhan along with him.

Kishore's friendship with Narasimhan grew as they worked together. Narasimhan was a simple man from a simple background. He continued to work with Railways late into his life and was a Class I officer at the time of his retirement.

Narasimhan was amused by how Kishore kept his finances and managed his expenses. Despite his ordinary salary, Kishore made it a point to send some money to his parents every month and after accounting for his daily needs, was still able to save. Narasimhan himself would often run out of money a few days before the payday and would have to borrow money. He used to joke, 'If someone sees your bank balance, they will think that you go around robbing banks! How are you able to save money when others are perennially falling short of funds?'

The Chief Electrical Engineer was an intelligent and kind man, and his words echoed in Kishore's mind long after he had left the Railways. '*Take a decision on the spot, do not procrastinate!*' his boss would say, asking Kishore to follow his gut. '*Your first thought is always the right thought. Even if it is not right, you have a chance to correct it later.*' Or, '*Don't be scared of anyone. Do not fear the consequences. Share whatever is being churned in your mind.*' These principles resonated well with Kishore. His simple, down-to-earth nature and values imbibed from his parents, helped Kishore adopt these teachings. This imbibed virtues of integrity and honesty in him, that remained with him all through his career.

From 1964 to 1971, Kishore had a great run in his first job. He also enjoyed living by himself, and soon developed a passion for reading. While the Railways took care of his *earning*, he still had to worry about his *learning*. He had been deprived of this opportunity in his childhood, but now Kishore would not miss a chance to buy or borrow a good book. He would spend whatever little money he could on books. He was exposed to the Ramakrishna Mission and its activities and it was there that he read the complete works of Swami Vivekananda. Much like Mahatma Gandhi and Vinoba Bhave, heroes of his childhood, Kishore now became a huge fan of Swami Vivekananda. He imbibed many of his teachings in his daily life.

Due to acute poverty in his childhood and youth, Kishore did not have many options for recreation or entertainment. He had relied on long talks with his friends when it came to knowing about movies and music. His only source of music had been an old radio that his father used to occasionally play in their home.

After he joined the Railways, with the newfound freedom of time and spare money to spend, Kishore built interest in movies. He followed films and film music, enjoyed watching movies of actors like Raj Kapoor, Rajendra Kumar, Guru Dutt in the 1950s to Dev Anand, Rajesh Khanna and later, Amitabh Bachchan in the 1960s and 1970s. Kishore was so impressed by

Dev Anand that in 2007, he bought the actor's autobiography, and read it in one sitting. Despite his strong views against smoking, Kishore was enamoured by the Dev Anand song, '*Har fikr ko dhue mein udata chala gaya* (I made all my worries blow up in smoke),' and would quote it often throughout his life.

While his stint with the Railways had many advantages and he was learning a lot, there were challenges as well. He often came across instances of corrupt practices. The numerous instances of open theft of property, even from coaches parked in the yard, horrified him. In the tendering process, there were leaks of confidential information, modification in requirements to suit certain parties and bribe accepted to get a particular bid selected. As Kishore was not willing to compromise on his integrity and honesty, he would not encourage any malpractice or wrongdoing. But he was not in a senior position, so the impact he could make on stopping or even reducing these malpractices was limited. His unwillingness to toe the line on corruption was proving to be a hurdle in his promotion.

◆

His old friend in Bombay, Krishnakumar had joined his family business straight after college and was doing well for himself. During one of his work trips to Bombay, Kishore discussed his problem with Krishnakumar. After Kishore updated him on the progress he had made in the Railways and the new work that he was involved in, Krishnakumar himself broached the topic: 'It's been more than five years in the Railways. In corporates, they say if you have been in one job for five years, you'll remain there forever. But I'm not sure if it's true in Railways as well.'

'Yes, while it's true that these five years have been good for me, I am not sure if I want to continue with the Railways forever.'

'Is something bothering you?'

'The issue is corruption. The way they expect bribes for

every purchase we make. The superiors expect us to toe the line, as if it is ingrained in us. I have grown up with ethical and moral values, my conscience does not permit me to support these practices.'

For anyone else, this would have been hard to understand. But Krishnakumar had known Kishore since his childhood. During their school days, even when his friends offered to pay for his meal at the canteen, Kishore would not like it, so Krishnakumar knew where he was coming from.

'Hmm. I do understand your challenge. But before you quit, you need to have an alternative job.'

Kishore thought about it before he replied. 'Yes, and for the new job, I am flexible about the location. My parents are getting old, I would prefer to be in Bombay, but I will be fine with any other city in West India. I've had to travel a lot to meet them when in South.'

Krishnakumar knew the owners of a company in Bhopal, Permali Wallace Limited. Permali was a leading manufacturer of laminates and insulators in India. They were looking for an Electrical Engineer in their Purchase department.

On Railways, he advised Kishore: 'if you do not feel comfortable, make a demand they cannot accept and leave. With such a stellar record, you can negotiate for a better salary in your next job.'

Kishore found this advice to be quite straightforward and he decided to pay heed to it. Krishnakumar assured Kishore that he would forward his résumé to Permali.

On returning to Secunderabad, Kishore told his manager that he needed to move closer home, as he had to take care of his ageing parents. Kishore was certain that the manager's area of influence was limited to Southern and Eastern Railway, and he would not be able to facilitate Kishore's transfer to the Western Railways, a completely different division. Comforted by this thought, Kishore initiated discussions with Permali

Wallace for a potential role.

Ironically, when Kishore finally decided to quit the Railways, he learnt that his manager, on the basis of his excellent credentials and track record, had been able to not only push the case for his transfer to Western Railways with a posting in Bombay, but also secured a promotion for him. However, Kishore had made up his mind and stuck with his decision to move on. This ended his glorious seven-year stint with the Indian Railways.

The Railways awarded its employees with three special passes to make a journey anywhere in the country. Kishore had for long wanted to travel across the country. He decided he would take a month's leave, and use all the passes. He took trips from Kanyakumari in the south, to New Delhi in the north. The second pass he used to travel from Madras all the way to Ahmedabad in the west. Subsequently, he went to Rameswaram, Madurai, and Pondicherry (Puducherry now) in the south before heading back home to Bombay.

5

GOODBYE BACHELORHOOD

Love is but the discovery of ourselves in others,and the delight in the recognition.

—Alexander Smith

On 3 April 1971, Kishore was married to Lata Parmanand Popat (Lata). It was quite a dramatic affair with lot of twists and turns, not unlike a Bollywood movie.

On 24 March 1971, Kishore reached Bombay at the end of his month-long journey across India, just in time to attend the wedding of Jyoti Suchde, a friend of his cousins, Charulata and Kokila Barai from Madras. Jyoti Suchde was also Lata's cousin brother. This was the first connection between Kishore and Lata. The day after the wedding, Kishore met some of the other family members, and Lata's name came up during some of the discussions.

Almost immediately, Kishore's details were shared with

Lata's family in Sion. Their first impression was positive, and Lata's family decided to set up a meeting at a bookstore run by Kishore's uncle, N.M. Thakkar & Company.

The person representing Lata's family was her aunt, Niti Jasraj. Kishore was surprised to see Niti there. Niti was Kishore's classmate from school. The moment Niti heard about Kishore, she wanted to meet him. As all of this happened extremely fast, Kishore had had no time to arrange for good clothes for the occasion. Kishore hastily borrowed a blue shirt from his brother, Bharat, known in the family for his great sense of fashion.

There was a hue and cry about Kishore's beard, which by now, was thick and black. Beard was not in fashion in those days. He assured them he would trim it in time for the wedding.

Horoscopes were shared and matched, only after the confirmation of the same did Kishore get the opportunity to speak to Lata. They met up at the Cream Center restaurant in Chowpatty and talked for half an hour.

Lata had many concerns, and so did her family. The beard was the least of the problems. When considering Kishore's financial status, the small house of her potential in-laws worried her. Unlike Lata, who grew up in an upmarket suburb of Bombay, Kishore lived in a small house in one of the remote suburbs, Kandivali, and there were six people living in that house. Once Lata was assured that she would not be living in that house as Kishore was to relocate for a job in Bhopal, she was not so worried.

Lata's father, Parmanand Popat was suffering from Parkinson's disease, hence her uncles and aunts were involved in the groom selection process. One of her uncles, Suryakumar Chottai, was also Kishore's classmate from school and strongly supported the match. Finally, the pandit chipped in with the decisive opinion, assuring them that the horoscopes pointed that the match was "*one in a million*".

Now that all the worries had been allayed, the wedding date had to be fixed. Kishore mentioned that he had to leave for Secunderabad on 4 April, which was less than a week away. It was decided that the engagement would take place on the 30th of March and the wedding would be held on the 3rd of April. Lata and her new husband would leave for Secunderabad the very next day. It was his last week in the Railways. They were married with great pomp and joy, and travelled quickly to Secunderabad using one of Kishore's special first-class passes.

Lata barely spent any time in Secunderabad, while Kishore wrapped up his stint with the Railways and said heartfelt goodbyes to his colleagues. Soon after, the couple boarded the train for Bhopal for Kishore to join his next firm, Permali Wallace.

The staff at Permali was surprised to know that Kishore was married. One of the managers, Mr Gandhi, who had interviewed him as a bachelor a month ago, wished him luck, and confirmed that the company accommodation would be provided for the newly-weds. So, comfortable arrangements were in place for them when they reached Bhopal.

Once Kishore and Lata had settled down, the Permali family invited them over for dinner. Tara Bhabhi, wife of the MD, Ranjeet Bhai, was very impressed with Lata and casually enquired whether she would be interested in working with them. Lata was not surprised that she was offered a marketing role. After her BSc, she had worked with a furniture retail showroom. She had a knack for sales and marketing, but she was new to the city and recently married, so she politely declined the offer.

Finding a house proved challenging for the couple. Despite Kishore's decent salary, the rents were high, but Lata did not even blink before offering her own savings. They moved into a new house in TT Nagar. Very soon, Lata was pregnant. The pregnancy was complicated, as were all the customs and rituals that they were expected to follow, but Kishore and Lata were fortunate to have helpful neighbours in the colony.

The nation, however, was in turmoil. There was yet another war with Pakistan. The Indo-Pakistan War of 1971 was a military confrontation between the two countries that occurred during the liberation war in East Pakistan from 3 December 1971 to the fall of Dacca (Dhaka now) on 16 December 1971. Pakistan's preemptive aerial strikes on eleven Indian Air force stations led to the commencement of hostilities with India and its entry into the war of independence in East Pakistan on the side of Bengali nationalist forces.

The war lasted just thirteen days, during which, Indian and Pakistani militaries simultaneously clashed on the eastern and western fronts. The war only ended after Pakistan signed the Instrument of Surrender on 16 December 1971 in Dacca, marking the formation of Bangladesh. It is estimated that members of the Pakistani military and supporting Islamist militias killed between 300,000 and 3,000,000 civilians in Bangladesh. As a result of the conflict, almost 8 to 10 million people fled the new nation to seek refuge in India.

It was in such a challenging environment that Kishore and Lata's daughter Manali was born on 6 January 1972.

6

SETTLING DOWN

People are always blaming circumstances for what they are. I don't believe in circumstances. The people who get on in this world are the ones who get up and look for the circumstances they want, and if they can't find them, make them.

—George Bernard Shaw

On 12 April 1971, after a seven-and-a-half-year stint, Kishore left the Indian Railways to join Permali Wallace in Bhopal, the capital of Madhya Pradesh. It was not an easy decision to make and his seniors at the Railways did not want him to leave. However, they respected his decision and gave him a warm farewell.

Kishore had taken a bold but risky decision. He had had a promising career with a lot of opportunities for growth in the Railways, but as it was a government-run organization, there were challenges—the politics and slow decision-making bothered Kishore. Permali, on the other hand, was a private organization, and it did not have the same issues of hierarchy and their management was progressive and encouraged independent action.

After thorough consideration, the management at Permali placed Kishore as the Head of Purchase and Stores Department.

This was a challenging assignment for Kishore. At that time, Permali purchased goods worth lakhs of rupees every month, including many new products. The Stores section that he was to lead, included recording and auditing, which was a completely new field for Kishore. He had six months to scale up his knowledge of the products and understand the complete auditing process. As the Head of the Department, he had to make sure exactly what his team was handling.

Kishore also had to get familiar with the vendor supplier ecosystem outside of Permali. The items to be purchased were supplied by multiple vendors. Understanding the strong points of each vendor, evaluating their products, negotiating for the most viable rate, making the vendor agree to a time schedule that aligned with the production schedule and finally ensuring that the products were delivered on time, were all responsibilities that he and his team were tasked with. In the 1970s, Bhopal was still a small city and bulk of the purchasing was to be made from vendors in other cities including Bombay, Calcutta and Madras. Hence, he had to make frequent work trips.

Back then, the company collaborated with Permali Gloucester in the United Kingdom and many components were imported from there. It was the period of Licence Raj in India and there was a long process involved in getting approvals for every single purchase. The job of the purchasing department extended beyond product development as it also included procurement of all raw materials, parts and even construction material for the factory expansion.

Kishore felt that it was a thankless job. While there was little appreciation for right decisions, umbrage would result on faulty purchases. This tough working environment early on, prepared Kishore for the long association with Permali.

Working for a private firm had its advantages and Kishore enjoyed the freedom to make decisions and execute them. He placed orders to the tune of two crore rupees, which was a big amount in those days. Changes took place in his personal life as well. Manali was growing up fast, and they had a second child. Their son, Hetal was born on 27 May 1974. With two kids and household chores to manage, Lata had her hands full.

They decided to leave the company flat, very close to the Permali factory. The Vitthaldas family, owner of Permali Wallace, also lived in the neighbourhood. The owner's children were of the same age as Hetal and they would often meet in the evening to play together. While Hetal enjoyed their company, the staff members would treat Hetal differently—even discriminating between them. When Hetal mentioned this to Kishore, and on further advice from some of his colleagues, Kishore made the decision to move to a house in Arera Colony, another locality in Bhopal.

In summer of 1975, as he was well settled, instead of travelling to Bombay during the summer, Kishore decided to call over his parents and sisters Renuka and Jyoti to Bhopal. As the eldest child he was cognizant of his duty to his parents, even while settling down with his new family. While they all were in Bhopal, Kishore fulfilled a long-standing wish of his parents. The entire family made a memorable trip to North India, visiting Haridwar, Rishikesh, Mussoorie, Delhi, Agra and Mathura.

Having had a deprived childhood himself, Kishore did not want that for his children. Bhopal was a small town, so it did not have the best stores for books or stationery. He would carry a long shopping list during his work trips to Delhi and Mumbai, making sure his children got the best. Whether it was a hockey stick or a table tennis racket, he would bring for both his children, without playing favourites. Kishore would get multiple copies of good books, to gift to his nephew and Hetal's friends as well, inculcating the habit of sharing in them.

When deciding what school to join, the kids were adamant on their choice. Hetal was clear that he would only study in Campion, while Manali wanted to go to St. Joseph's Convent. These were the two Jesuit-run schools in the city, and considered the best for boys and girls respectively. Moreover, Manali and Hetal's friends all studied there. This put their parents in a quandary.

'Lata, we will need to talk to the kids and convince them to consider other schools,' Kishore told Lata after returning home one evening. Tired as he was from the day's work, he knew he could not let the matter linger.

'I know why you are saying this, but they go out to play with their friends and get all the information from them. They cannot be easily convinced,' replied Lata, who was also aware that Kishore's salary was not sufficient for the family's many growing expenses.

'Then we will have to make more compromises on our spending,' Kishore said.

Lata, being the efficient housewife that she was, made the necessary calculations that very night. The next day, they initiated the admission process for both their kids and got them admitted into the most prestigious schools of Bhopal, where they studied from Grade 1 to high school.

In 1980, Permali suffered a major crisis. Their main raw material, veneer, was supplied from their own unit in the southern state of Karnataka. However, their supplies had now been exhausted and they had to urgently look for alternative suppliers. Kishore decided to look for alternative sources in the North East, so he spent six months travelling through Guwahati (Assam) and Tin Sukhiya (Nagaland) in search of an appropriate supplier. Kishore was forty-two, when he took his first flight from Calcutta to Guwahati. This heralded yet another exciting phase of his life.

7

THE FAMILY MAN

Regret for the things we did can be tempered with time; It is the regret for things we did not do that are inconsolable.

—Sydney J Harris

Kishore, being the oldest of four siblings, had willingly taken up the responsibility of earning and taking care of his family. Whether it was funding his own Engineering, or sending money home while working as a bachelor in the Railways or while as a family man when in Permali, Kishore was always there to support his family.

It had been easier when he was a bachelor, but after his marriage and with two fast-growing kids, his family expenses had increased. But Kishore was committed and was fortunate to have very understanding employers at Permali, managers who would accede to his requests for leave and advances whenever there was an emergency.

Kishore had seen his parents struggle to make ends meet throughout his childhood. He had observed that despite their dwindling finances, his mother would make personal sacrifices to feed the family. As he was now settled and leading a decent life in Bhopal, he wanted to give back to his parents.

When travelling to Bombay for work, he would procure best quality grains and pulses from Bhopal and take for his parents. Lata would even make *sabu dana papad* and potato chips in large quantity for Kishore to take for his parents. His friends in Bhopal often remarked that Kishore did more for his parents in Bombay, than what they did for their own in Bhopal.

In 1981, Kishore received a proposal for his sister, Jyoti's marriage. It came from Mafatlal Trivedi, an old business associate and also a good friend. He shared details about Narendra Thakkar, a young man working as a marketing manager for an auto parts company in Ahmedabad. Kishore and the family approved the match, and the marriage was solemnized in 1982.

But all did not go well with the marriage. Narendra was a troubled man, suffering from mental illness so severe that it took a toll on Jyoti. Despite going through the physical and mental trauma, she continued to believe that Narendra would get better, and hence did not disclose the issue to her parents and brother.

Within first year of marriage, Jyoti was pregnant, and Narendra's condition had not improved. It was through one of their neighbours that Mangala Ben finally got to know about the issue. She immediately called up Kishore and the family decided to take a firm stand on the matter. With Jyoti being pregnant, their first priority was to minimise her mental trauma.

Kishore decided to bring Jyoti back to Bombay to stay with her parents. Permali was expanding at the time, and as part of his responsibilities, Kishore would travel to meet various suppliers across the country. He tried his best to spend a few extra days whenever he was touring Bombay. Kishore reassured his father, and acted as the head of family by providing immense emotional and financial support to the family. In Bombay, Kishore also sought counsel from his old friend Pravin and they evaluated various options to resolve the matter.

Jyoti soon gave birth to a beautiful girl child, Khyati. Within a few years of their separation, Narendra passed away because of a heart attack. While saddened by the development, Jyoti knew that she now had to look ahead in life. She decided to focus on Khyati's education and Mangala Ben's health, which had deteriorated of late.

Kishore supported Jyoti financially as she had decided not to remarry. Khyati was a bright and intelligent child and Kishore took up the responsibility for her education. He would get gifts for her whenever he would travel to Bombay. He encouraged her to concentrate on her studies and provided her with spiritual guidance. Khyati did not disappoint, and she went on to get a PhD in the United States. It was Kishore who did the due diligence, managed her wedding ceremony and did her *Kanyadaan* (giving away of the bride) during Khyati's wedding.

Vinodrai, now in his sixties, having retired some time back, was keen to take up a small job himself. After what Jyoti had undergone and the family having additional needs, he wanted do his bit. Kishore spoke to Pravin, and arranged for a job for him in a small firm in South Bombay, Trinity Pharmaceuticals. He was supposed to manage the operations of the pharmacy shop in the absence of the shop attendant.

After a few months, the long arduous train commute from Kandivali to South Bombay was becoming tough for Vinodrai. Late one evening, on the way back from the store, he met with an accident when a scooter hit him as he was crossing the road. He had fractured his leg and was rushed to the well-known Bombay Hospital nearby. When the news reached Kishore he took a train the same night to Bombay. After a couple of days of recovery, he was brought home to Kandivali. While Kishore told his mother that he would take care of the financial impact, he knew Jyoti now had the additional responsibility to take care of their father

In the meantime, Jagadish too had got married and had shifted to another house in Bombay. Kanak, his wife subsequently gave birth to two sons, Mehul and Kinjal. Kishore's younger sister, Renuka, had decided to pursue a career in teaching, and also took care of their parents.

Sometime in 1984, Jyoti, who was pursuing a career in nursing, was practising in a small town in Gujarat—Virnagar. Khyati was only a year old then. It had become difficult for Renuka to take care of both the parents and hence Jyoti requested Vinodrai to come over to Virnagar and live with her. While there, Vinodrai had a paralytic attack and was bedridden. The left side of his body was completely paralyzed.

Jyoti got him admitted to a hospital in Virnagar. After about a week, their uncle and Jaisukhram Bhai (grand uncle) visited the hospital to see Vinodrai. Jaisukhram Bhai was part of the caretaker family of the Jalaram Bapa Trust. (*Jalaram Bapa was one of the Gods the family worshipped.*) Vinodrai was a long time devotee of Jalaram Bapa. All through his adult life, though never well off, whenever he had any spare cash, Vinodrai would donate some money to the Jalaram Bapa Trust in Virpur. Kishore and Jagadish would not like this. They would complain to Vinodrai, but he would not listen to them. Jaisukhram Bhai was aware of Vinodrai's devotion for Bapa. After meeting Vinodrai and talking to the doctors about the treatment, Jaisukhram Bhai left to return to Virpur by the evening train. Before leaving, he quietly left an envelope with a large sum of money under Vinodrai's pillow; the amount was far bigger than the meagre amount that he would have sent as donation. When Kishore heard about the money, he was full of guilt; Vinodrai's strong faith and allegiance in God had been aptly repaid.

Vinodrai, meanwhile, needed to remain in the hospital. Jyoti had not envisaged the situation and needed help to take care of Vindorai. She wanted him to be moved to Bombay, where he would receive better medical care. Jyoti called Jagadish, who came over to spend a few days with Vinodrai. Jyoti hesitated to speak to Kishore; at the time Kishore was extremely busy with work in Bhopal, making frequent trips to northeastern part of India.

Ultimately, when Vinodrai's health did not improve, Jyoti asked Kishore for help. Kishore was in Assam at that time and he instantly took the first flight back to Bhopal. From Bhopal, he took a bus to Indore, and then a train to Virnagar via Ahmedabad. He reached Virnagar late the next day. During the trip, he realized he had not thought about how to get Vinodrai—in his paralytic state—to travel with him.

The next morning, Vinodrai was overjoyed to find his eldest son by his bedside.

'Kishore! *Tu avi gayo? Arey Wah!*' (Kishore, you have come, very good!) He exclaimed, his eyes welling.

He told Kishore that he was keen to return to Bombay. He wanted to be there in time for Renuka's wedding, which was scheduled in a month's time.

Once they reached Bombay, there was a long discussion. Mangala ben said she would not be able to take care of Vinodrai alone as Renuka was getting married soon. Kishore had to make an urgent work trip to Assam. So, it was decided that for a month till the wedding, Vinodrai would stay with Renuka and Mangala Ben. When Kishore would be back in Bombay for the wedding, he would consider taking Vinodrai to Bhopal.

When Kishore and Lata reached Bombay for the wedding, Lata was concerned about Vinodrai being brought home to Bhopal. She was worried about taking care of her paralytic father-in-law by herself, especially as Kishore travelled frequently for work. But Kishore was able to convince her after a long discussion. She alone proceeded to Bhopal the next day.

A few days later, Kishore began to make plans to take Vinodrai to Bhopal. This was around the time when Prime Minister Indira Gandhi had been assassinated by her bodyguards in New Delhi, which had led to increased tension all across India.

The situation in the country was very grim. As the bodyguards who killed Mrs. Gandhi were Sikh, the Congress leaders, angered by this dastardly act, decided to direct their anger towards the Sikhs, questioning the integrity of the whole community. There were reports of barbaric acts being committed in various parts of the country, especially in Delhi. Bombay also had a lot of Sikhs. Being a metro, acts of violence were also expected in Bombay. Sikhs in Bombay were also known to drive auto rickshaws and taxis. There was a fear of them being tortured and/or killed. The other possibility was many Sikhs, fearing attack from their neighbours, might try and flee Bombay by train and head to Punjab. This meant possibility of them being attacked on the train. Kishore was advised not to travel under such circumstances. As most of this was just rumour, Kishore decided to take a chance.

By sheer coincidence, when Kishore mentioned his travel plan to Pravin, his old friend offered his mother's wheelchair for Vinodrai. However, it had to be picked up from his house in Walkeshwar, the farthest end of South Mumbai, an additional fifteen minutes ride further from Bombay Central Station.

Kishore and his ailing father got into a rickshaw from Kandivali, and subsequently hailed a taxi from Bandra. As they started from Bandra, it was already 3:30 p.m. The train was scheduled to leave at 4:30 p.m. Kishore hurriedly explained to the taxi driver that they needed to go to Walkeshwar, pick up the wheelchair and then proceed to Bombay Central station.

The taxi driver obliged and rushed, and they reached the station with the wheelchair by 4:15 p.m. Kishore was aghast, and wondered how he would carry Vinodrai to the platform and board the train. The driver pointed out that it was time to use the wheelchair.

The range of emotions going through him at the time—worry, fear and anxiety, perplexed Kishore. He felt like crying at his misery and laughing at his absentmindedness at the same time. Finally, with support from the driver, they were able to board the train just in time. After all the drama that ensued till that point, the rest of the journey was rather uneventful, and they safely reached Bhopal the next morning.

◆

It was the evening of 2 December 1984.

It had been a month since Vinodrai had moved to his son's house in Bhopal. Vinodrai was in recovery and needed constant care and attention. After an early dinner, the kids played cards and spent time with their Dada (grandfather). Thereafter, everyone went to bed by 10 p.m.

Kishore was awakened very early in the morning by noises outside. He stepped out and saw people moving around in cars, on scooters, bicycles and even bullock carts. Kishore quickly returned inside and switched on the radio. He heard an announcement about a catastrophic accident—earlier that night 30 tonnes of methyl isocyanate (MIC), a highly poisonous gas, had leaked into the atmosphere from the storage tank of a pesticide factory owned by Union Carbide (UCC), a Dow Chemical company. Kishore again went outside and a man informed him that thousands of people in the vicinity of the factory had died due to the gas leak and those who survived were complaining of a burning sensation in their eyes. The man also spoke of a more recent and deadlier second leak.

The Sonpals lived approximately fifteen kilometres away from the factory, and had it just been the four of them, Kishore would have probably not been as worried, but he had to take extra precautions for his ailing father. Kishore immediately spoke to Mr Sacarda, GM in Permali Wallace, who advised Kishore to bring his family over to their house, which was on the outskirts of the city. They packed all urgent belongings, including his father's medications, and left in their Fiat car. To protect themselves from exposure to the poisonous gas during the trip, everyone covered their mouths with a wet cloth or towel.

They soon found out horrifying details of the world's biggest industrial disaster. The poisonous gas spewed out of the factory and spread more than 40 square kilometres; and people at a distance of five to eight kilometre downwind were the most seriously affected and for them Bhopal become a gas chamber that night. It was widely believed that had it not been for the two lakes of Bhopal, which came in the way of the moving gas cloud and neutralised it, a tragedy of much greater proportions could have taken place.

Luckily for the Sonpals, the winds had not been strong that night and the gas did not reach the locality where they lived. After spending a few hours at Mr Sacarda's house, it was clear that the news of a second leak was a rumour, and the Sonpal family decided to return back home. It was a sombre realisation for Kishore, as he had narrowly escaped death once more in his life, and this time around, so did his family.

◆

After this harrowing experience Kishore had to make a two-week trip to Assam. Fortunately, by this time, both Manali and Hetal were enjoying the company of Dada. Vinodrai loved playing cards with them. Although he would lose in *Dhagla Bhaji* (a popular card game), he would enjoy watching his grandchildren laugh when they beat their Dada. He would also narrate many mythological tales, including stories of Lord Rama and Lord Krishna. These stories were more informative than what they learnt at school. Lata was able to adjust well with her father-in-law, especially because he was a simple man with few needs.

On a particular day during the Assam trip, Kishore was looking forward to the taxi ride in the evening back to his hotel in Guwahati, hoping for a nice sumptuous dinner and some sleep after a tiring day of negotiations with suppliers. Upon reaching the hotel, a telegram was handed over to him by the manager.

'Father has hurt his leg, suspected fracture. Please come home.'

Kishore reached out to his manager, Mr Sacarda, and updated him on the development. He immediately proceeded to fly back home. Vinodrai's happiness knew no bounds when Kishore walked in; he forgot about his broken leg and was about to stand up, when Kishore held him back.

Kishore had already consulted a good orthopedic at a nearby hospital. But Vinodrai indicated that he would not go to a hospital. Kishore was perplexed. He knew the family shared a traditional distaste for hospitals, but he had not expected such stubbornness. The next day, Kishore explained the problem to the doctor, who agreed to treat Vinodrai at home.

A plaster was cast at home and Vinodrai's leg had to be supported with a home-built traction system for twenty-one days. He was completely immobile and needed round-the-clock care. Lata was amazed by how Kishore managed to take care of his father, occasionally getting up in the middle of the night and at odd hours to heed to his every request while continuing his demanding job at Permali.

The doctor called it a miracle, when within twenty-one days, the fracture had healed completely. After a few days of regular physiotherapy and exercise, Vinodrai was able to walk again. He had recovered through sheer will power.

A couple of days later, sometime in the afternoon, when Lata went to Vinodrai's room to check on him she noticed he was not there. She immediately called Kishore at his office. He shared that his father had mentioned about wanting to go to the Birla Temple, but Kishore had not anticipated he would go without telling anyone. He comforted Lata and told her that he was coming home right away.

After they had waited anxiously for two hours, a very tired Vinodrai walked into the house, barefoot.

'Where had you gone, Bhai? And where are your *chappals* (footwear)?' Kishore questioned angrily as Vinodrai handed him some *Prasad* (temple offering).

'I had gone to the Birla Temple to pray. After offering the prayers, as I was about to leave the temple, I noticed that my chappals were gone. Either they were stolen, or a dog must have taken them away. So I walked back barefoot.'

Kishore took some time to comprehend what his father had done: having just recovered from a leg fracture, he walked seven kilometres to the temple and then walked back home barefoot. Kishore had no heart to probe further and helped Vinodrai get back to his room to rest.

However, Kishore's love and devotion for his father could not prevent the eventuality. Six months after moving to Bhopal, Vinodrai died of a heart attack on 11 May 1985. Kishore considered himself fortunate that he got a chance to serve his father in his last days. He lit the pyre and bid farewell to his father, one last time.

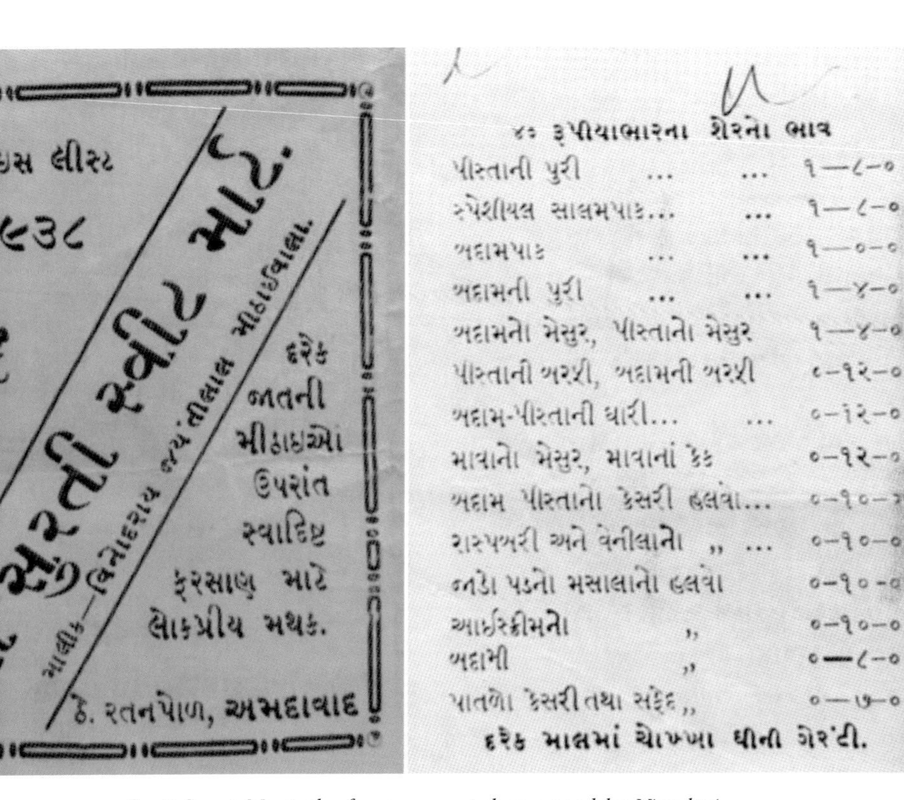

Surti Sweet Mart, the famous sweet shop owned by Vinodrai

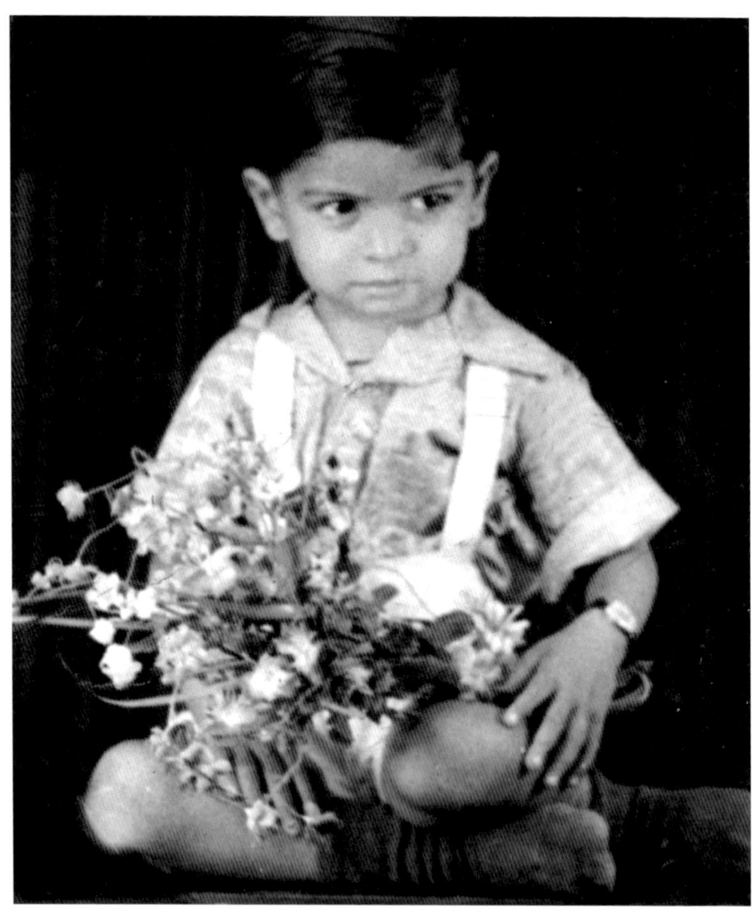

Kishore in his childhood, 1942

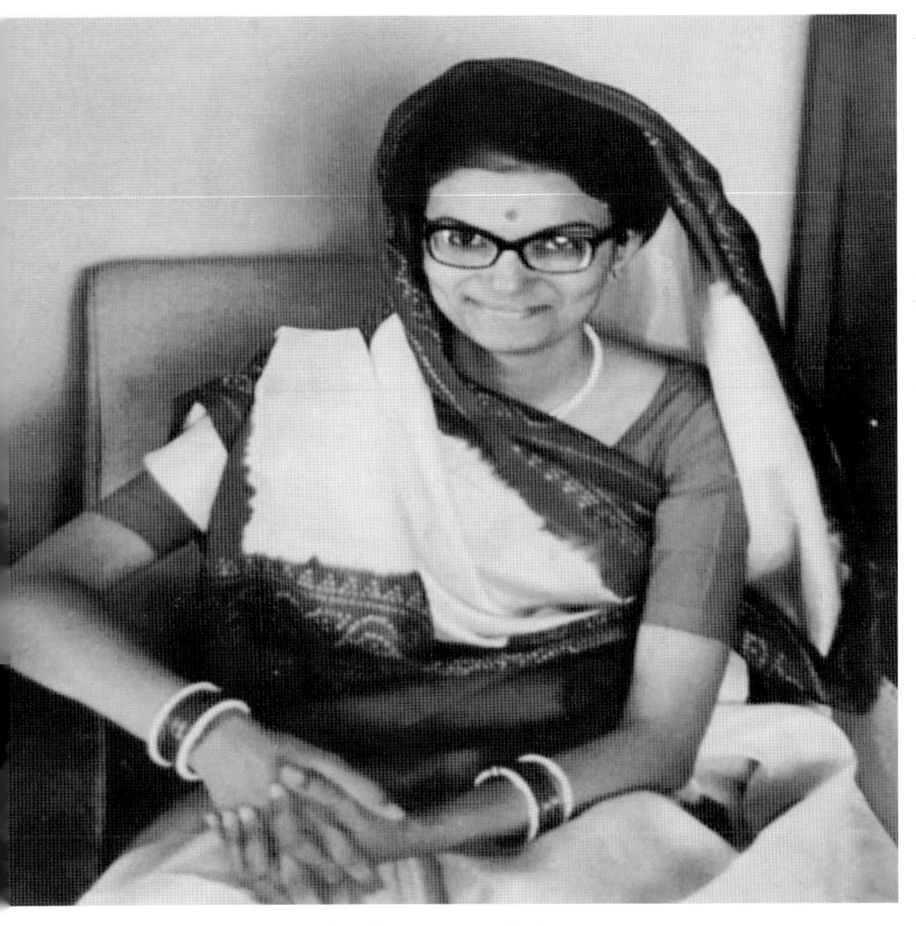

Kishore's gorgeous wife, Lata

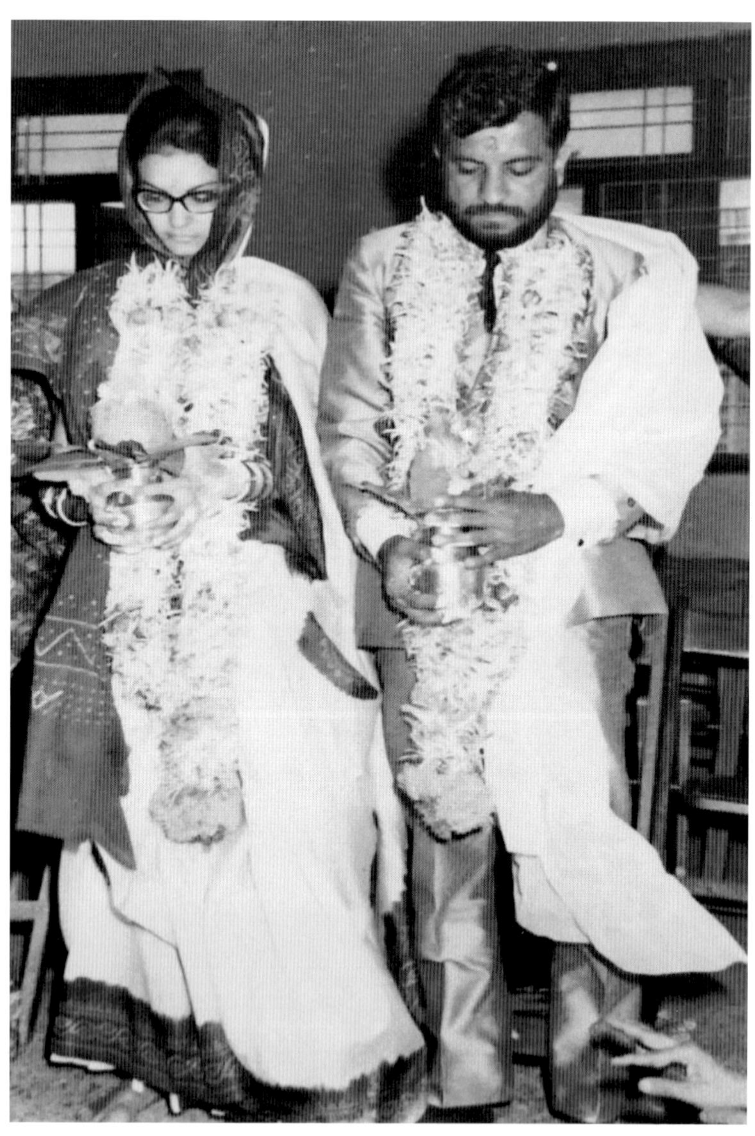

Kishore's wedding, 3 April 1971

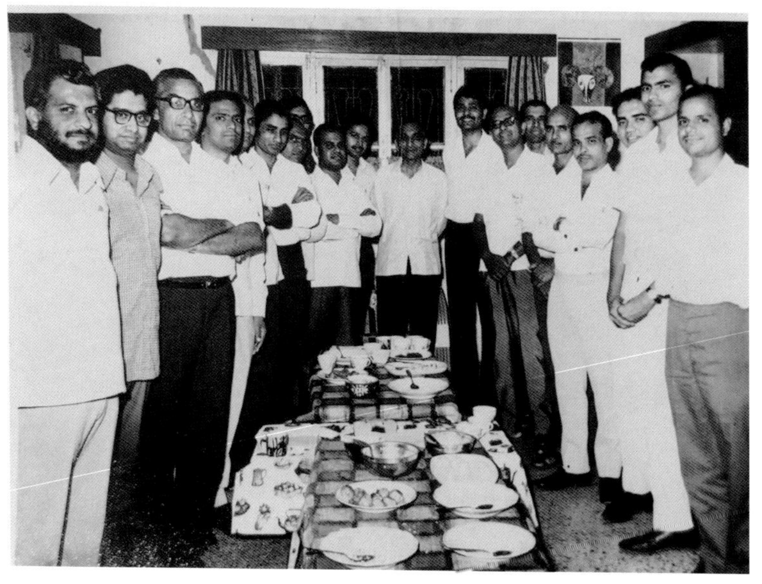

Kishore with the Permali team in 1971

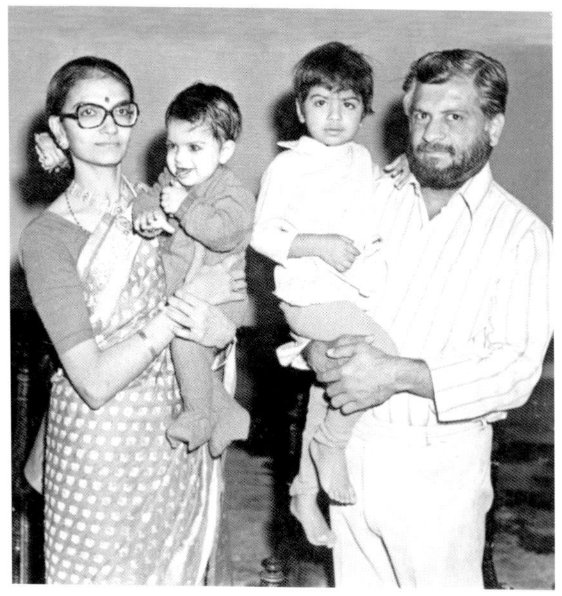

Lata, Hetal, Manali and Kishore in 1975

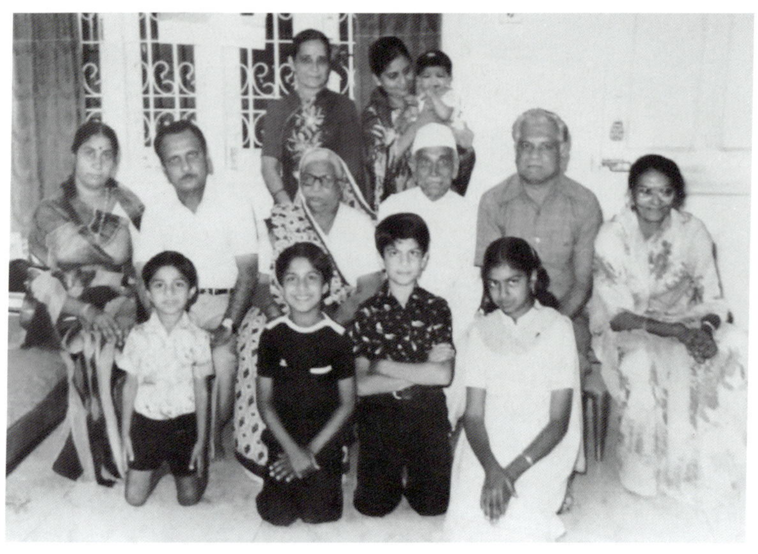

The Sonpal family in Bhopal in 1981
Top row (L-R): Renuka, Jyoti, Khyati.
Middle row (L-R): Kanak, Jagadish, Mangala Ben, Vinodrai, Kishore, Lata.
Front row (L-R): Kinjal, Mehul, Hetal and Manali

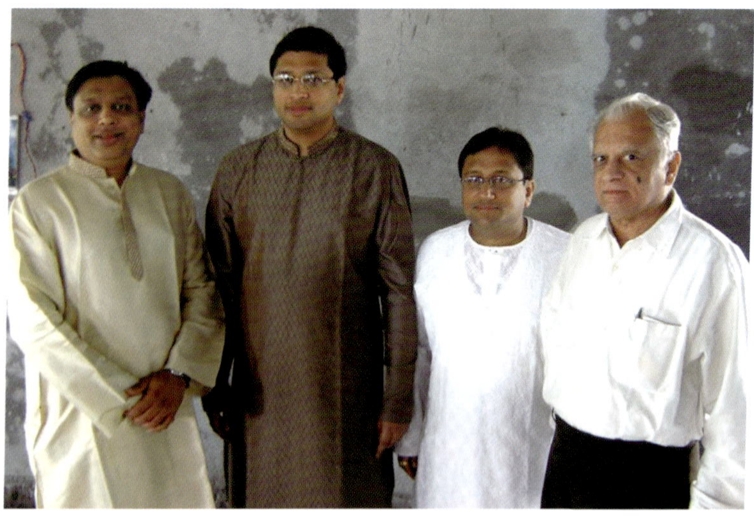

The Mangal team in 2005: Hiten, Nayan, Dhiren and Kishore

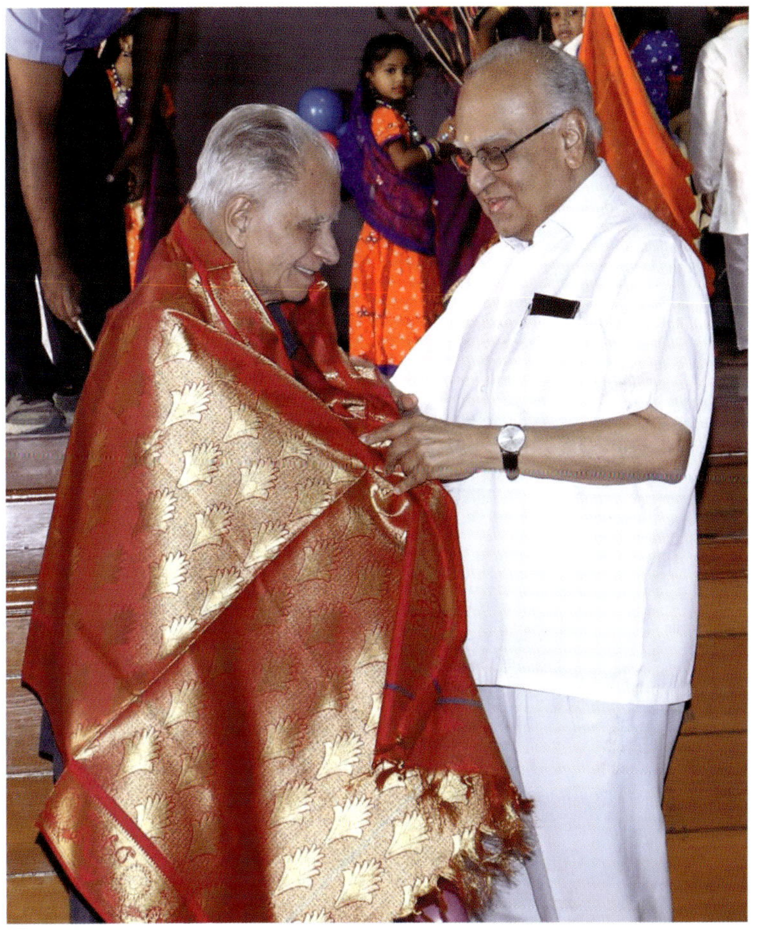

Kishore being felicitated by the Chairman of Bharatiya Vidya Bhavan for 10 years of service in March 2019

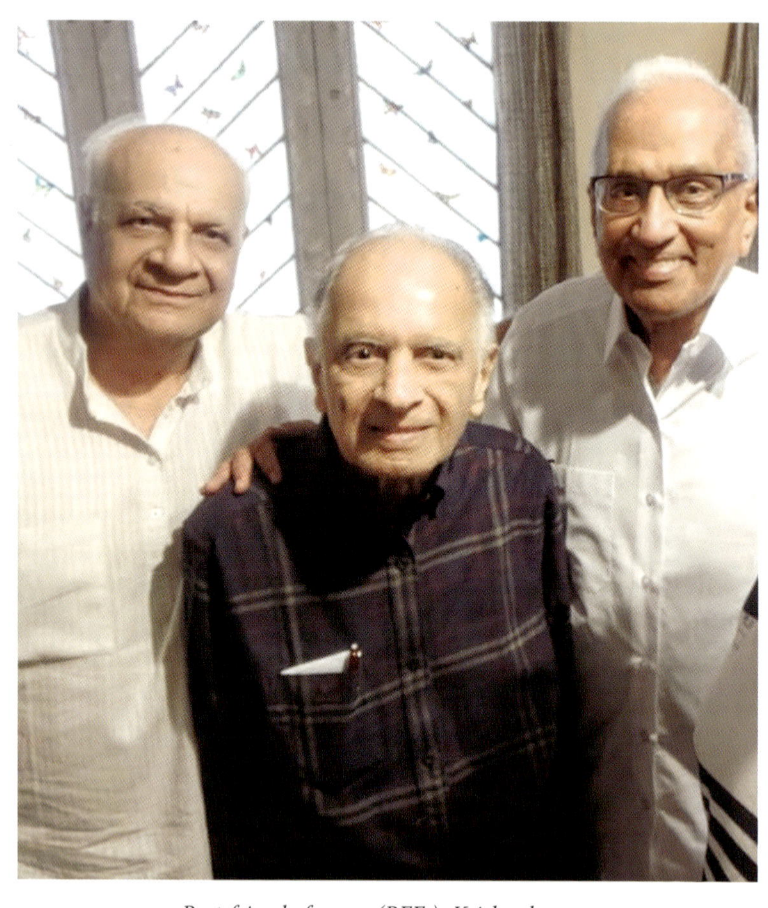

Best friends forever (BFFs): Krishnakumar,
Kishore and Pravin celebrating 70 years of friendship in 2020

8

NARROWLY ESCAPING DEATH

> *Our very survival depends on our ability to stay awake, to adjust to new ideas, to remain vigilant and to face the challenge of change.*
>
> —Martin Luther King Jr.

20 October 1980. It was a cold winter night in Bhopal.

'Don't worry. I will call you once I reach Kandivali. You are used to my routines by now!' Kishore assured Lata as he boarded the autorickshaw. He was to travel to Bombay by train, on the *Punjab Mail* scheduled to leave Bhopal Railway Station at 8:00 pm.

'Please take care and do have the *theplas* (a type of chapatti famous in western India) that I have packed.' Lata replied as Kishore got into the rickshaw. 'And I have informed Hema that you are travelling in F1 and you will meet them in their S2 coach. She is travelling alone with Premal and Pinky, and

Bakul Bhai wanted to make sure you can watch over them.'

'Of course, I will meet them in the train, not the platform, it's simpler that way. Incidentally, Dhiru Bhai's (A family friend) wife and daughter are also travelling in the same coach. His one month-old grand-daughter is also with them.'

'I'm surprised they are travelling with such a young child,' Lata said.

'So was I,' Kishore added, placing his bag into the vehicle. 'Apparently they have a religious ceremony. They have had a child after sixteen years of waiting, so it is a special event.' With this, Kishore finally bid his wife goodbye and asked the driver to proceed to the railway station, a fifteen-minute drive from their home.

Upon reaching the station, Kishore boarded his coach without much trouble. The rush was less than usual, and it pleased him. *Crossing over to the S2 coach inside the train would be easy*, he thought.

The train left Bhopal station precisely at 8 p.m., and Kishore settled down. He opened the pack of theplas, and noticed a bottle of buttermilk also packed for him. Once he was done with dinner, Kishore walked towards the S2 coach to meet Hema and the kids. They were very old family friends of theirs.

Hema was glad to see him. Dhiru Bhai's family was in the same compartment, and had already been introduced. The kids were playing with the baby and there was a cheerful atmosphere in the coach. A berth was vacant in the same compartment, so Kishore decided to shift.

'I will come back around 10 p.m. with my bag. I hope you will have finished dinner by then,' Kishore told Hema. Hema was grateful. Kishore rejoined them at about 10:30 p.m. The train had halted at Itarsi station, which was a major junction on the route. The halt was long. With Hema and kids and Dhiru Bhai's family well settled, Kishore decided to sleep.

Within fifteen minutes, Kishore woke up. A loud noise

resounded through the compartment.

BANG!

Before he could get what was going on, he toppled from his upper berth and fell with a thud on the floor of the train. A couple of suitcases fell on him and he groaned in agony. There was commotion as the whole coach toppled and landed upside down.

What followed next was a spate of screams, chaos and wails. All hell broke loose. People were thrown off of their berths and were falling atop each other.

Somehow, Kishore got his bearings and looked around. Fortunately, one of the train guards was close by and he held out his hand to help Kishore get up.

'Babuji, there has been an accident,' the guard told Kishore as he reached the door of the coach. Pitch darkness had descended on a moonless night, and there was zero visibility in the coach. Kishore had travelled a lot and was well versed with the railways due to his last job and realized that it was a head-on collision. The coaches in front would have borne the brunt of the damage, and their carriage, the seventh from the engine, was not that badly impacted. But opening the door proved difficult.

A half-hour passed in complete confusion and chaos, and Kishore helped and comforted the others while waiting. Some of the people were injured but not badly hurt. They heard voices outside. The rescue team from Itarsi had come.

They learnt that the train had collided with a stationary goods train. Their coach had gotten detached due to the impact and had fallen headlong into a ditch next to the track. As it was the outermost track and the coach toppled outwards, it was not in line of other oncoming trains. The first three bogies were badly smashed, and the telescopic effect had made them pile on top of the engine.

The rescue team was prepared for action and they slowly

helped people out. Kishore ensured that Hema and family and Dhiru Bhai's family members were first brought out of the coach. Fortunately, the baby had been sleeping with her mother, who had clung tightly to her and they were both safe.

After about fifteen minutes of waiting near the tracks, a rescue train came to get them back to Itarsi station. It was then that Kishore noticed his torn shirt. He was still in his pyjamas that he had changed into before going to sleep. Ironically, some lady raised hue and cry about her missing slippers and this brought some much-needed laugher among the survivors. A member of the rescue team lent her a pair of shoes and consoled the lady. The train was to be pulled back to Itarsi by an alternative engine subsequently. While a train was being arranged for Bombay, Kishore, along with most of the co-passengers, preferred to go back to Bhopal.

On the homeward journey, they got more details of the accident. Apparently, the driver of the train had missed a red signal. Of the total 731 passengers in the train, there were about 138 passengers in the first four coaches, which were the worst impacted. Among these 138, 16 people had died on the spot and three more succumbed to their injuries later in the hospital.

The third coach from the engine of the train had buckled and bent into a U-shape; its shell consequently collapsed and distorted, before the whole structure was atop the locomotive. A shiver went down Kishore's spine when he realized what he had just escaped. *The third coach from the engine was F1. He had narrowly escaped death.* The extraction of the injured and the dead from the coach was a challenging task, and it called for tremendous patience, care, ingenuity and improvisation on the part of the team. The last of the injured was spotted at 9 a.m. the next day under all the metal and debris.

Due to presence of large quantity of debris and the flammable structural composition of the collapsed coach itself, a fire broke out in one of the coaches, and it took a long time to put off. Fire fighters provided assistance with commendable alacrity and the fire was eventually put out, but only after it raged for two whole hours. Many of the bodies were charred beyond recognition.

Kishore, along with some other harried passengers, had missed getting their names registered in the list of survivors. They were busy trying to get back to Bhopal.

In the meanwhile, news of the accident had reached Bhopal early in the morning. As he was on a business trip, Permali management was concerned and they quickly sent someone to Itarsi to check on him. There were no quick means of communication available then, and all the information was unreliable.

As Kishore had shifted coaches in the night, his name did not feature among the survivors of the first-class coach. So the Permali team enquired whether a man with a thick black beard had been seen. They were exasperated when they could not get any information on Kishore.

Kishore and the others managed to get a bus and reached Bhopal at 10 a.m. After ensuring that Hema and the kids reached home safely, Kishore, with his bruised arm and torn clothes, proceeded towards his home in Arera Colony.

While most of the dead bodies had been recovered and the process of identification was on, some of the coaches had been badly damaged, so these would take more time. The team from Permali proceeded to Bhopal to update the management, and more importantly, to inform Lata.

'What? What happened to you?' Lata was aghast to find Kishore in tattered clothes at the door. His arms and legs were bruised.

As Kishore came in and sat down, Lata got him a glass of water. Once settled, Kishore narrated the story of the accident and how they had managed to get out of the coach and had made their way back to Bhopal. She sat with her face in her hands. She had been busy with the morning chores and had not switched on the radio, and had no idea about any rail accident.

While Kishore was narrating the details, the doorbell rang. Lata opened the door to find a couple of people from Permali. They were about to share the unfortunate news with her when they noticed Kishore, bruised, but alive in his own living room!

Kishore explained again. Hetal and Manali were happy to see their father safe; they were much too young to gauge the gravity of the accident that their father had narrowly escaped.

Only when Kishore narrated how he had shifted to second-class coach, that his colleagues from Permali finally understood the source of confusion.

'Now it's clear. We checked and rechecked in the list of survivors from the first-class coach. Not only was your name not there, none of your co-passengers remembered seeing you there at the time of the accident. We were perplexed!'

The Permali staff members were relieved to see Kishore safe and sound, and soon left. Kishore took a long shower. With prayers, he thanked God for having saved his life.

The next day at the office, the Permali MD, Ranjeet Bhai, suggested that Kishore should go on a pilgrimage. Kishore and Lata went on a trip to Nathdwara in Rajasthan and Virpur in Gujarat to pay homage to the gods. Incidentally, adventure and misfortune followed them there also as Lata's gold chain was snatched amidst the huge crowd that thronged the Nathdwara temple.

In Virpur, Lata's uncle made a suggestion that Kishore agreed to. In acknowledgement of the new life God had given him, Kishore shaved off his beard that he had kept for almost twenty years. Lata, who had always disliked the beard, even before their marriage, was happy to see it go.

9

THE GLORY DAYS

The method of the enterprising is to plan with audacity and execute with vigour; to sketch out a map of possibilities and then to treat them as probabilities.

—Bovee

The 1980s was a good decade for the Sonpals: Kishore felt quite settled in Bhopal, both the kids were studying in the best schools in the city, Lata had adjusted to managing the house, and he was able to fully attend to his work and career.

While in town, Kishore had a set routine. He was always the first to wake up. He would meditate, go for his morning walk and then proceed with the daily chores. On days when Lata could not wake up early, Kishore would be the one to wake up the kids for school and would even prepare and pack their lunch.

As the children grew, so did their knowledge of the world. Kishore had never been exposed to western music, as English music was known then, but he got a new cassette player for the kids. Next, the excited kids needed someone to introduce them to the popular singers. Kishore spoke to a few of his colleagues and arranged for cassettes of popular singers including Michael Jackson, Stevie Wonder and Madonna. He was very particular that his own disinterest in anything should not mean his children be deprived of the same.

Lata took the lead on engaging the kids in extracurricular and sports activities. As Kishore had little time to spare, she took upon herself to teach the kids how to ride a bicycle. They bought a cycle much bigger for their age and without any training wheels, so they would learn it the hard way. She would take the kids on her Luna, a popular two-wheeler in those days, for swimming lessons as well. While Kishore was not into movies, Lata loved watching them. She would occasionally take the kids to the theatre over weekends. Hetal and Manali would look forward to these outings. When television sets were introduced in the country, the Sonpals bought a Keltron, a black and white television brand in 1983.

Lata, who had worked for a short time before marriage, yearned to work again. In the mid-80s, with Manali and Hetal in middle school and able to manage their studies, Lata had time for herself.

Instead of a typical 9-to-5 job she was interested in entrepreneurship. Though she had weak eyesight, she enjoyed stitching. One of their earliest purchases was a stitching machine. So, when it came to starting something on her own, she decided to convert her passion into profession. She observed the increased sales of stitched garments at that time. The 1982 Asian Games, hosted in New Delhi, had generated a sports boom in the country. And more players meant increased sale of garments of stretchable material.

Through a common friend, Lata signed up for an entrepreneurship development course and religiously attended all the lectures. During the course, she met a few women, who were planning to set up their own stitching unit at home.

'You want to set up a stitching unit, here? Inside the house? Is there enough space for it?' a surprised Kishore asked Lata when she told him about her plan. While he had encouraged Lata to sign up for the course, he was certainly not expecting this! With his limited knowledge in running a business, he was not sure how he would be able to support her.

'Our guestroom is empty, so I can use it for my stitching unit. We need to go to Indore to check the machinery. We can be profitable in six months,' Lata replied confidently.

And profitable they definitely were. Starting off as a hosiery unit making vests on contract, she went on to make t-shirts and clothes for babies. Eventually Lata had her own shop to display and sell her garment range. From a normal housewife, Lata became a full-fledged businesswoman, while still managing the duties at home.

Kishore had a dream to have his own house. But owning a house was expensive, hence he had been saving up for the same. In the mid -1970s, his colleagues had suggested he buy a plot and build a house himself.

In the 1980s, the state government floated a scheme to allocate a large piece of residential land for plots of different sizes and then sell the plots individually. The plots were categorized based on income groups—Low, Mid and High Income groups. Kishore was allotted a MIG plot in an upcoming part of Bhopal, Gautam Nagar, close to BHEL (Bharat Heavy Electricals Limited) township.

Two years after the project was initiated, the contractor assigned to build the houses left the project midway and absconded with the capital invested by the plot owners. It was a huge setback for Kishore. While other owners contemplated legal proceedings, Kishore was not willing to wait for his dream home.

A while ago, Kishore had been associated with the construction of Permali House, the official residence of the Vitthaldas family. This experience would now come handy for him, right from finding another contractor to getting suppliers for the construction material. Lata also chipped in by going to inspect the project daily. Kishore was very clear that he would get the best possible material that he could afford for his dream house. He even travelled to Delhi to get light fittings and tiles.

Kishore also built a passion for Indian classical music. The Vitthaldas family was very fond of classical music and had set up Abhinav Kala Parishad, headed by Mr Tated. The Parishad invited prominent artists to perform in the famous Rabindra Bhawan, a prestigious auditorium in Bhopal. Right from the tabla maestros, Ustad Alla Rakha and Zakir Hussain; sarod genius, Ustad Amjad Ali Khan; sitar player, Pandit Ravi Shankar, to ghazal legends, Chitra and Jagjit Singh, Bhopal was host to all of them, thanks to Abhinav Kala Parishad and Permali. Kishore and family got to hear them all.

One chilly Friday night in October, Lata and the kids got off the Lambretta scooter as Kishore parked it in the parking area of Rabindra Bhawan. They were looking forward to hearing the magical duo Pandit Shiv Kumar Sharma and Ustad Zakir Hussain.

Mr Tated greeted them at the entrance with a look of concern. 'Mr Sonpal, you are aware of the rules of these functions. You know Ranjeet Bhai is strictly against allowing kids into the auditorium,' he said to Kishore. 'They spend a lot to watch these artists in complete silence. Your kids may not like the show and might disturb others.'

Kishore knew his kids, they were well behaved. He

confidently walked up to Ranjeet Bhai, who was talking to a few guests in the front row and made his request.

'Sonpal, promise me that the moment your kids make any noise, you will leave the auditorium. If they do NOT make any noise, then I will personally invite them for the next event,' Ranjeet Bhai said to Kishore.

Fortunately, both Hetal and Manali were quiet throughout the evening and left an exceptionally good impression in the mind of the Permali Management.

Kishore instilled ideals in his children in many similar ways. One such plan was to impress upon them the importance of being financially prudent. To teach them the habit of saving, he decided to give Hetal and Manali a major responsibility.

'From this month onwards, I will not be handing over the money for household expenses to you,' Kishore informed a completely shocked Lata in 1987. Lata was aware that expenses had to be better managed as they were moving to a new property, but she was unsure about what Kishore just told her.

'Relax,' Kishore smiled. 'I am not suggesting any further cuts. I am only suggesting that instead of you, I will hand over the money to Manali and Hetal. They will be accountable for keeping track of all the expenses that you make to run the house.'

Kishore intended that they take charge of all the accounts and make their own budget. 'Right from the maid's salary to money for vegetables, you will ask them for the money. They must make a note of all expenditure. At the end of the month, they will provide us with a summary on all the expenses under various headings.'

Lata thought about it for a moment and then smiled. She immediately understood Kishore's plan. Although she had grown up in a well-endowed household, after fifteen years of marriage, she had become astute in spending. Kishore would now teach his children to do the same. She agreed immediately, adding, 'While I am certain Manali will manage it well, as she is in the 10th grade, Hetal will need some time to learn.'

Kishore had already considered this, and said, 'I have a different task for him. From now on, he will be going to the bank for menial tasks like updating the passbook or depositing cheques. If the amount is small, I also want him to withdraw cash. Even before they know how hard it is to make money, let them feel the experience of dealing with a nationalised bank holding your money.' The couple agreed, and they explained it to a surprised Hetal and Manali that evening.

The next day, the staff at the Bank of Maharashtra branch in the neighbourhood was thoroughly amused to see a thirteen-year-old boy in t-shirt and shorts at the cash counter to withdraw 200 rupees! This was an early lesson in financial management and banking and it proved very crucial for Hetal later in life. By the time he was on his own in college, he could manage his finances far better than his friends, and early in his career, he was also able to make smart investment decisions.

Kishore decided to realise yet one more of his childhood dreams. He had always wanted to have a stamp collection. He signed up at the local post office to get all the stamps and the first day covers issued every month to be delivered home. Hetal was quick to adopt this hobby and along with coins, they together build a vast collection. Kishore would happily observe as Hetal would proudly show his collection to his friends and they would exchange stamps. Kishore even introduced his nephew Mohan in Kolkata to philately; whenever he would travel to the city for work, he would get stamps for him and review his collection.

And Kishore loved food. Not only did he enjoy sumptuous meals, he was quite skilled at the nuances of cooking. He had learnt when helping his mother at home and while working with his father in the family business. When visiting relatives, he had a wish list of what he looked forward to eating. Kishore would do justice to everything that would be served to him! With family history in the food business, he wanted his children to experience all the good food. Bhopal had few good bakeries, so whenever he would travel to Delhi for work, he would make sure to get cakes and pastries from Nirulas.

One day, during a regular meeting at work, Permali MD, Jaisinh Bhai, noticed that Kishore was not drinking his tea. When he enquired, Kishore informed that he had given up drinking chai.

'Oh, how can you do that, Kishore Bhai? You can give up anything else, but how can you give up chai? *Chah chodi deso to jeevso kevi reetie* (How will you live, if you give up tea?)?' Jaisinh Bhai remarked, and the room split into laughter.

Chah, which means tea in Gujarati, in Hindi means desire, a major driving force in one's life.

The secret to Kishore's success was his honesty, integrity and strong resolve. His predecessors never lasted long in the company. All of them were easily enticed into accepting bribes from the vendors for placing large purchase orders. As the head of the department, he placed orders for crores of rupees and it was normal to expect 10 to 20 per cent as commission. When Kishore faced this situation the first time, he found a smart solution. For an order of Rs. 100,000, where the vendor was willing to offer Rs. 20,000 as commission, he would ask the vendor to include the commission as a discount in the pro forma invoice. The company was surprised to get such high discounts from vendors who had stuck to their quotes for decades. The company gave him a raise to thank him for his negotiating tactics. The elements that led to his predecessors losing their jobs helped Kishore get him his promotions.

Kishore faced the same challenges during the Licence Raj, as he earlier faced in the Railways; grafts, bribery and corruption. Each new challenge rattled him and shook him to the core. Each time he would question the meaning of his own existence.

But in Permali, he was able to face that same challenge bravely. Integrity was the lifeblood of Permali. The management emphasized that they would not compromise on this principle. Mr Gandhi, the Sales GM, often said, '*Even the simple wooden pencil provided to the employee is company property and one is not supposed to take it home.*' In his charismatic style, Mr Gandhi once told Kishore, 'Your cabin, Mr Sonpal, is made of glass. Everything that you do inside is clearly visible to the people outside. The smallest stone of allegation of any wrongdoing that hits the cabin will shatter the glass, and also your image. So please keep that in mind.'

Kishore recalled his words often, especially when dealing with issues of integrity.

Ranjeet Bhai used to tell Kishore, 'Kishore, don't do anything that will make us lose our sleep. We can buy anything in this world, but we cannot buy sleep.' Encouraged by the honest work culture, Kishore's ethical realm grew larger.

In another instance, Kishore observed that when submitting medical bills for reimbursement for tax benefits, people would often submit fake bills. However, if someone was fortunate to be healthy and wished to submit bills for healthy products like Bournvita (a famous chocolate drink) or Chyawanprash (healthy food), it was disallowed by the company policy.

'So, you actually want me to fall sick and then claim reimbursement for medicines instead of being reimbursed for items that keep me healthy?' a confused Kishore asked the head of HR. True to the sprit of Permali, the management acknowledged his point and amended the policy to allow certain items to be considered for reimbursement.

For official travel by train, the company provided Kishore first class travel allowance. However, it was possible to travel in second class and claim first class fare for reimbursement and pocket the difference. Kishore would strongly advocate his team members to desist from such a practice. Kishore observed that life is far from perfect and everything is not in black and white. There are shades of gray in many cases and one needs to have an astute sense of foresight and judgment to see through and take the necessary steps that best suit the situation.

After almost two decades with Permali, Kishore was happy and his profile continued to grow. Kishore had surprised everyone by continuing for so long. While there were enough reasons to continue, Kishore felt that he was missing out. The children were almost ready for college. But life in Bhopal had its shortcomings, with few opportunities for professionals. Kishore wanted his children to be exposed to many career choices and not be limited by those in Bhopal.

Kishore was fifty-two years old. It was the age where he could still take risky decisions. He felt that he still had a few more years left in him to take bold, aggressive steps to enhance his career and change the fortune of his family.

India meanwhile was in a crisis at that time. The balance of payment problem that troubled the government in 1985 had blown into an economic crisis that shook the country in 1990. The government was close to defaulting, and its central bank had refused new credit. Foreign exchange reserves had reduced to the point that India could barely finance three weeks' worth of imports. It had to pledge 20 tonnes of gold to the Union Bank of Switzerland and 47 tonnes to the Bank of England as part of a bailout deal with the International Monetary Fund (IMF). Most of the economic reforms were forced upon India as a part of this bailout.

In response, the finance ministry led by the then finance minister, Manmohan Singh, initiated the economic liberalization in 1991, with the support of Prime Minister Narasimha Rao. The reforms did away with the Licence Raj, reduced tariffs and interest rates and ended many public monopolies, allowing the automatic approval of foreign direct investment (FDI) in many sectors. These same reforms, by the turn of the 21st century, enabled India to progress towards a free market economy, with a substantial reduction in state control of the economy and increased financial liberalization.

On 12 November 1991, based on an application from the Government of India, the World Bank sanctioned a structural adjustment loan meant primarily to support the government's programme of stabilization and economic reform. This specified deregulation, increased FDI, liberalized the trade regime, reformed domestic interest rates, strengthening the capital markets (stock exchanges) and initiating public enterprise reform (selling off public enterprises). Now businesses like exports, that enabled foreign exchange to come into the country, were being encouraged. Direct support was provided for entrepreneurs willing to set up manufacturing units. Kishore felt that as a career change it would be good to be part of a venture that was export-oriented, to benefit from the huge wave of liberalization that had stormed the nation.

At the end of 1991, Kishore moved out of Permali and joined Mangal Exports in Mumbai. His job was to be based in South India, to purchase textile material. Hiten Dalal, son of his childhood friend, Pravin Dalal, had started Mangal Exports. While his family continued to live in Bhopal, Kishore moved to Coimbatore, famously known as the Manchester of South India, to start his new adventure with Mangal Exports.

In a glowing tribute to Kishore at the time of his leaving Permali, the GM, Mr Sacarda, said:

Mr Sonpal was the head of the purchase department in Permali Wallace Ltd. He used to control all types of stocks for the factory, including raw materials, finished products, working materials and factory equipment. He was an outstanding engineer with a Bachelor of Engineering in Electrical Engineering. He provided exemplary service for fifteen years at Permali Wallace. He had amazing engineering insights and problem-solving skills while being extremely enthusiastic with utmost dedication to his work and colleagues. A hardworking senior executive, an honest leader, he always sought to improve the company with his creative and positive attitude. He was always happy and smiling!

As a senior executive, he was in charge, taking full accountability and responsibility of anticipating the needs for different kinds of raw materials to ensure that the factory operated efficiently. He could anticipate problems ahead of time and predict the needs of the factory to ensure smooth operation. During his 15 years tenure, there was never a day where the production at Permali suffered, a glowing testament to his management style and engineering excellence.

10

GREENER PASTURES

You have to leave the city of your comfort and go into the wilderness of your intuition. What you'll discover will be wonderful. What you'll discover will be yourself.

—Alan Alda

Early in June 1990, Kishore's old friend Pravin called him. He had a proposal. He wanted Kishore to consider a job change and join his three sons, Hiten, Dhiren and Nayan, in their newly launched textile exports business, Mangal Exports.

Pravin had had a long and successful trading business and had since retired. Hiten, his eldest son was based in Mumbai, and had already dabbled in different businesses but with little success. Dhiren, the second son, had started a stationery business, which had not yielded good results. Nayan, the youngest, was completing his MBA in New York. While he was keen on working with his brothers after graduation, he wanted to stay in the US.

Pravin felt that Kishore, with his vast experience, would be able to guide the three brothers, while actively contributing as a team member. Pravin's elder brother, Vasant Bhai, recommended Kishore. Kishore was able to procure a special elaichi, a rare product from a remotely located supplier for him, accounting for the minutest details. Pravin too highly valued Kishore's acumen and he suggested that Kishore meet Hiten in July and discuss the opportunity.

Kishore indicated he would love to consider the option seriously. As he kept the phone down, he reflected on his good fortune. Twenty years ago, Kirshnakumar, one of his closest friends had suggested the Permali job, and now it was his other friend, Pravin, doing his bit. He flew down to Hyderabad in the subsequent week and met Hiten. The textile industry in India was fairly large at the time, producing a wide range of products. Right from bed-sheets to tablemats, towels, and napkins the industry catered to the needs of customers globally. It was famed as a cottage industry and was a source of employment for thousands of workers, delivering precious foreign exchange for the government. Especially after the recent economic liberalization, there were more and more textile units being set up across India. However, Mangal's initial focus for exports was only cotton napkins and tablemats, catering to customers who supplied these products to the large restaurant industry in the US.

Based on preliminary research, Hiten had contacted a few agents, suppliers and manufacturers and fixed a few meetings. As Kishore hailed from an electrical engineering and technical background, the subject of textile was new to him. However, he had perfected the art of purchasing and knew the nuance of trade. His traits of accounting for details, open-mindedness and having a calm demeanour under pressure was brought to good use.

The typical process involved meeting a supplier and asking

them to show their product range. Then they were given the sample provided by the customer/export house/agent and asked to make a matching sample for quality inspection. Based on the quality of the sample and negotiations, the order would be finalized. Even in a simple product like a table mat, right from quality of fabric, shades of the colour, yarn used, etc. lot of points were evaluated. The quality of the yarn and the weaving had to be judged and the price had to be extremely competitive. Even after selecting the right product factors like cost and timely delivery were very important.

After meeting with vendors in Hyderabad, Hiten and Kishore had a series of meetings in Bangalore (Bengaluru), the Garden City of India, known in those days for its beautiful gardens and pleasant weather. From Bangalore, their next stop was small city of Chennapatnam, where they went by road.

Chennapatnam, a city 100 km from Bangalore, is the largest base in India for wooden toys and other wooden products. The Mangal team met suppliers for napkin rings. Apart from the design, the key evaluation criteria included the product finish and colour fastening. After a productive day in Chennapatnam, Kishore and Hiten got back to Bangalore.

Carrying on with their hectic schedule, they had a train to catch the same night to Erode, on the way to a major industrial town in Tamil Nadu, Karur. On reaching Erode early morning, they found that the only way to reach Karur was by bus. Extremely tired by then, they spent two hours in the Erode railway station retiring room waiting for the bus to Karur. Even before starting, Kishore was living the challenging life of a start-up.

In Karur, they were better prepared. Hiten had established contact with an agent who had worked out a plan for meetings with various suppliers and export houses. Karur being one of the largest textile export hub in the early 1990s, the Mangal team had planned to spend the maximum time in the city.

Apart from the generic considerations involved in choosing the right textile supplier, the type of weaving done is very important. Only 3 to 5 weavers in the city had acceptable capabilities; access to good quality and regular supply of yarn were the other factors to be considered. Cotton was procured from North India, which then had to be processed and spun. Two types of yarn were popular, reel and hank yarn. Hank yarn was used for hand dying—its 100-150 threads bundled together in a typical way. The colour, design, size, quality, etc. needed to be confirmed before approving the product.

After Karur, their next destination was Cananore. There they met another agent who had lined up supplier meetings for the Mangal team. Kishore observed that though there were fewer suppliers in Cananore, the quality of their products was much better.

Finally, taking a detour from Erode again, Kishore and Hiten completed their eight-day trip. Kishore took a train back to Bhopal and Hiten returned to Bombay. Once he was back home, Kishore prepared a detailed report, summarizing their research work and minute observations from all the meetings. As he did not have access to a typewriter, he wrote the report by hand.

Based on the review of the report and detailed discussion among the three brothers, it was decided that Hiten and Nayan would travel with Kishore to the South again in December 1990. Nayan was in his final year of MBA, and would have his winter break in December. The second trip to the South was similar to the first one, and this time Kishore impressed the two brothers with his immense knowledge and understanding he had built about the business.

While considering the role, Kishore noted that communication would be a problem, since he did not speak any of the South Indian languages, especially Tamil. The other challenge was the heat—South India was hotter and drier than Bhopal. Even in the month of July, the temperature would sour to mid-forties.

During the second trip, Kishore's base location was discussed extensively. Instead of Karur, Coimbatore was preferred as it was a much bigger city with good infrastructure, better connectivity and good weather. Situated at the foothills of the Nilgiris—the Blue Mountain range—Coimbatore seemed like a great place to live.

However, his children were still in school, so Kishore did not consider it appropriate to move his family to Coimbatore. He would travel back and forth between the two cities every two months. Finally, it was decided that Kishore would resign from Permali to join Mangal in Bombay in February 1991, right after Dhiren's wedding.

This was an interesting transition for Kishore. Unlike the Railways and Permali, which were well-established firms, Mangal was a start-up. And he would be joining as a founding team member, not an employee!

In 1991, Kishore was fifty-three-years old. Typically, entrepreneurs run start-ups in their early twenties. Also, Kishore was joining a start-up in an unknown sector, settling down in a new state, where he did not know the local language. He would be away from his wife and teenage kids. It was a very bold decision on his part. Oblivious to the challenges that lay ahead, the spirit of adventure and the opportunity to create something new drove Kishore.

After remarkable twenty years with the company, Kishore formally resigned from Permali Wallace Limited in January 1991. Mahesh Bhai in the Permali management team reassured Kishore, 'In case things do not work out in the new venture, the doors of Permali are always open for you. We would be glad to have you back.'

On 12th of February, Kishore flew down from Bhopal to Bombay to attend Dhiren's wedding. He met many of the suppliers and other businessmen during the wedding and thus started yet another important chapter of his life.

11

STARTUP AT FIFTY-TWO

We act as though comfort and luxury were the chief requirements of life. When all that we need to make us happy, is something to be enthusiastic about.

—Charles Kinglsey

The early days for Kishore in Mangal were anything but easy. He was constantly travelling from his home in Coimbatore to different cities: Karur, Erode, Chennimalai, Tirupur, Cananore, Bhawani, Bangalore and Chennapatnam. He had to regularly write detailed reports of the work he was doing. These were the days when instead of email, mobile phones and video calls, long distance communication happened through landline phones, fax and courier. Each day, Kishore would leave home early in the morning and return late in the evening. He got little time to relax.

Kishore took time to adjust to such a demanding schedule.

But he was driven by a powerful mind that ensured he was very disciplined. He inculcated the new schedule as a habit over a period of time.

The travel schedule that Hiten and Kishore had established during their initial visit in 1990 became a routine as the company expanded. During his visits from Mumbai, to smaller cities, Hiten would look forward to their 'after office' discussions with Kishore, in their hotel rooms. In these discussions, Mangal would take a back seat and they would discuss topics like culture, philosophy and family traditions. Kishore had a collection of stories from the Bhagwad Gita to share, and was well versed with the political and economic development in the country. Hiten would remember these meetings as 'Swadhayay' (Self Evaluation) sessions. Hiten's understanding of life improved through these philosophical talks. While Hiten would wake up late, Kishore would be up at five every morning. He would have completed his meditation, morning walk and reading of the newspaper by the time Hiten would join him for filter coffee.

Kishore enjoyed treating Hiten to typical South Indian meals for dinner, followed by his favourite Amul ice cream and coffee to wrap it up. During some of the longer trips, they would visit some of the famous temples in Palani and Chennimalai. Lata would join them on some of these trips.

On the work front, there was a new development. Though it was Kishore's job to meet prospective suppliers, a nominated agent was to be kept in the loop. The supplier finalization was not solely Kishore's decision, but would include the agent also, which led to confusion and delay. It was evident to Kishore that the agent was earning commission from the suppliers and that influenced his choice. However, the team in Mumbai was oblivious to this.

Kishore's travel itinerary included going to Bombay every month. The thirty-six-hour train journey meant Kishore was losing precious time in travel. As he stayed at Pravin's house during these trips, work was discussed with Hiten over lunch, dinner and all the way till bedtime. He was literally working for Mangal round the clock. Work had completely taken over his life.

However, the trips to Bombay also gave him opportunities to meet friends and relatives. He found little appeal in staying in fancy hotels and would rather invite himself to any of the relatives' houses all across Bombay. Their houses were small, but Kishore was always welcomed with open arms—not because he would bring expensive gifts, but, as he would share something far more valuable: his knowledge and wisdom. Apart from enchanting and amusing people with his palmistry and face reading skills, Kishore was a well-read man and loved to talk. Conversations would delve late into the night, on topics ranging from spirituality, education, science and culture.

The greatest challenge in export business is that if the final product is not of good quality there is potential threat of entire shipment being rejected by the end customer. Mangal's journey, unfortunately, began with such an order. The customer rejected the poor quality of a delivery and Mangal had to take the entire order back, thus incurring a major loss. They had to even bear the cost of getting the goods back to India. Like any other start-up in its early phase, this was a tough loss for Mangal. Kishore had given up a comfortable job and the three brothers had invested their father's lifelong savings into the business; there was no going back now. Pravin arranged to cover up for the loss of the order and Mangal survived the initial setback.

Kishore's work trips now also included frequent trips to Madras, where he was able to renew the old bond with his sisters, Charu and Kokila. His jovial and easy-going nature enabled him to make friends with Kokila's son, Munna and daughter, Yogini. Munna would often take him around in the city on his two-wheeler. Kishore's knowledge of palmistry, developed through intuition and books, made him extremely popular among family and friends. Women in particular were charmed by his skills and they would spend hours asking him questions on what their hands revealed. Most amusing were the bold predictions that Kishore could make about the future, many of which later turned out to be true.

By March 1992, at the end of the first financial year of Mangal, the business was not in a great shape. Kishore proposed some key changes, including removal of the agent, as he was confident about sourcing buyers directly. The change was approved. Business flourished and soon, Kishore suggested they set up an office in Karur and hire staff. Kishore finalized a few suppliers who were willing to work in the long run. He also expanded his network, and studied the nuances that impacted supplier performance: yarn, mill, colour, quantity, MOQ, order turnaround time, labour availability, labour absence, etc.

Kishore also explored another city Chennimalai, located in Erode district for suppliers. Chennimalai had good weavers, but they were not engaged in exports as yet. Kishore felt that they had the capacity and quality to service export orders at a much cheaper rate. The pricing was the most attractive bit about Chennimalai: it was almost a third of that in other cities. Kishore decided to give a vendor in Chennimalai a chance to work on a large order. While Kishore was confident, Hiten was uncertain about trusting a new vendor. Kishore decided to set up an office in Chennimalai to monitor the production locally. Ultimately, the local office in the city ensured that the suppliers were kept on their toes and they delivered the order on time.

Kishore now had to juggle time in multiple cities and between different product lines. He was involved in strategizing and ensuring quality, while accounting for on-time delivery. Many of these new suppliers had no experience, and did not have a thorough quality-checking process and they credited Kishore for helping them build their businesses.

As Kishore built the supplier channel in South India, Mangal sales began booming. In five years, the company's turnover increased from 0 to 5 crores. Having built a large supplier base for different products with multiple suppliers for each product, Mangal was able to get competitive rates and thus make good margin in every deal. Because of his negotiating and decision making skills, he was also involved in expansion of Mangal's Bombay office. Kishore led the development of supplier network in Surat and Ahmedabad as well. He even expanded the north Indian supplier market, setting up an office in Delhi.

Being in South, while further away from Bombay, Kishore had not forgotten his duties towards his sisters and Khyati. Whenever he would visit Bombay for work, he would make sure to meet them. After Mangala Ben passed away in 1992, Kishore encouraged Jyoti and Renuka to continue their jobs, as a nurse and as a teacher respectively and also for Khyati to continue her education. He was a constant source of motivation for Khyati and it was due to Kishore's continued encouragement that Khyati went on to pursue her PhD in the US.

Sourcing, building a network of suppliers, setting up offices, and recruiting people: Kishore had managed all these activities initially in the South and then in the West; now he did the same in North India. In exports, it is important to maintain a deep relationship with the supplier. While negotiating well to get the best rates, cordial relation also had to be maintained so that they do not collaborate with the competition. Textile exports was quite a competitive sector and other exporters and agents were always looking for new suppliers. Within the next two years, business from Delhi region grew to over fifty crores.

By the late 1990s, Kishore had made a name for himself in the textile industry. Apart from his enhanced acumen on the industry lingua, Kishore was also known for his strong memory; he recalled old incidents, names, relations, birthdates, anniversaries, as if they were imprinted in his mind. His memory helped him to surprise people on their birthdays. On one such occasion, Kishore surprised Chandrasekar, one of the leading suppliers in Chennimalai, by greeting him with a gift and some flowers. Chandrasekar himself had forgotten his birthday, and was moved when Kishore drove down from Coimbatore just to wish him.

In the late 1990s, Kishore was exposed to the teachings of Acharya S.N. Goenka and the famous Vipassana programme. Not only did Kishore himself go to Igatpuri for the ten-day course, he even convinced Mr Chandrasekar of Kaveri Textiles to come along. Such close collaboration between a customer and a supplier was unheard of in any industry.

Suppliers would proactively set up meetings with him directly to showcase their samples and manufacturing prowess. The moment Kishore entered a manufacturing unit; he was able to gauge product quality issue from a distance, when even the shop floor head would have missed the error. When it came to quality checks, Kishore often said, '*What you see may be false, what you hear may be incorrect, but what you observe by investigation will always be correct*.' This inspired many suppliers, and became their guiding mantra. Kishore became a mentor and guide even to his suppliers.

Kishore, due to his strong negotiation techniques, was always able to negotiate hard to make the supplier agree to the right price, but with little margin left for the supplier. However, he was warm-hearted and to compensate the supplier, he would award a few more orders where they could make a decent margin and reap volume benefit.

When he left Bhopal in 1990, Kishore had planned to return back and live in his own bungalow there after retirement. But after a few years in the beautiful city of Coimbatore, he changed his plan and decided to invest in a flat there. He purchased a flat in a prominent and green part of the city on Race Course road, called Raheja Enclave. Kishore used to commute via a public bus to see the flat layout and meet the builder. Later, he came to know that the builders were laughing about Kishore coming to buy a flat in the most prominent locality while travelling in a government bus. What should have reflected his humility was instead judged harshly. Little did he know then that this would become his home for next twenty-five years.

Manali was married in 1996, and she moved to Detroit, Michigan, US. Since Hetal completed his engineering in the same year and started working in Bangalore, Lata joined Kishore. With a heavy heart, the bungalow in Bhopal was sold off and the family was now settled in Coimbatore.

Kishore realized that he had been so engrossed in setting up Mangal's business that he had not taken any vacation for nine years. Therefore, in the year 2000, with Manali expecting her first child, Kishore took his first major holiday. He and Lata went on a three-week trip to see their newborn granddaughter, Ashka. True to his style, even during the vacation, he spent a week for Mangal's work. He visited Nayan's office in New York and met some of the key customers.

After the holiday, Kishore resumed work with renewed vigour. Demand for products from Panipat and Delhi had increased and Kishore had to travel more frequently. Mangal's product range had expanded, and the turnover in 2003-04 was almost 80 crores. While pleased with the growth, Kishore ensured that the company did not lose focus on the bottom line: how to reduce costs without compromising on quality, how to build stronger relationships with suppliers, etc.

During one of the trips to North India, Kishore got a call from Hiten, who said, 'Kishore Bhai, please meet the zip supplier. The cost of the zip is higher than what we planned and is impacting the cushion cover pricing.' Kishore assured Hiten he would look into the matter. Kishore reviewed the rates of various zips provided by the supplier and then met him.

'Bharat Bhai, emphasis on quality is important in exports. That's why you quoted the price for your best zip, which also is the most expensive. However, the zips are to be used for cushion cover and not for apparels. In case of cushion cover, Americans have a use and throw policy and the zips are used very few times.' Kishore explained tactfully.

The supplier got the hint and reviewed his supply chain and manufacturing data. He worked out a revised price for the zip. Everyone in Mangal was amazed with the negotiation; the reduced price allowed them to win a large order of cushion covers subsequently.

In 2004, Mangal received a large order from Walmart, and decided to go for in-house production/manufacturing. Kishore was not in favour of this decision, but the management considered it a natural step in backward integration to make a handsome profit from such a large order. Significant investment was made to procure land, building and set up the operation.

The constant travel across the country was taking a toll on Kishore's health. He had started working with Mangal in 1990, when he was fifty-two. But in 2004, he was sixty-six, and it was tough to keep the same momentum. Also, he was a stickler about his fasts. During Navratri, twice a year, he would diligently observe the nine-day fast and would not even consume coffee while spending long hours negotiating with vendors.

Over a period of time, Kishore had built interest in spirituality. His journey of self-discovery had started earlier in the 1960s, when he was exposed to the Ramakrishna Mission and teachings of Swami Vivekananda. In the 1970s, after he moved to Bhopal, he and his family became ardent believers of the Gayatri Sect and Acharya Shri Ram Sharma. Later on, in the 1980s, after a trip to Pondicherry, Kishore was enamoured by the talks of Sri Aurobindo and The Mother. The doctrine of purity and simplicity, so well depicted in the simple life in the city and in the workings of the Ashram, left a deep impact on him.

Kishore loved to share his wealth of knowledge with others. Whenever he would come across some good piece of writing or good thoughts, he would ask his secretary to type it out and fax it to others within Mangal, his suppliers, family members and friends. Not confident that people would buy the book he recommended, he would buy the books in bulk and gift them to people.

During 2007-08, the Indian textile industry was facing increased competition from China, and it was further impacted by the global financial crisis. Excessive risk-taking by banks combined with the bursting of the United States housing bubble caused the values of securities tied to the US real estate sector to plummet, damaging financial institutions globally, culminating with the bankruptcy of Lehman Brothers on 15 September 2008, and an international banking crisis. The crisis sparked the Great Recession, the most severe recession since the Great Depression.

This crisis greatly impacted Mangal's large customer base in the US and Europe. Even though the turnover increased to 120 crores, it grew difficult to retain customers who were constantly asking for lower rates. Within the new set-up, Nayan decided to look for textile suppliers in China for more competitive rates. With the resulting drop in demand, Hiten decided to tap the domestic market for sales, and a new brand Bianca was born. Dhiren decided to pursue his dream to create herbal products, forming the Herbal Hills brand.

Subsequently, Kishore decided to end his journey with Mangal after nineteen years with them in March 2009. Later the same year, Mangal's under-utilized in-house manufacturing set-up was also shut down. By December 2009, the three brothers formally disassociated their working arrangements and this led to closure of the Mangal business.

In the words of Dhiren Dalal

The striking quality of KVS was that he had a charming personality and would always try to touch your heart. He would make it a point to know about your likes, your birthday, etc. He would know someone very fast, in the first meeting itself.

My main learnings from KVS include:

- *On the topic of China, it was worth observing that people from all over the world approach the Chinese due to their low cost. No Chinese salesman is going out and selling in the world. That's the dominance of a superpower.*
- *KVS always tried to develop personal relationships with our suppliers by talking about their families, their likes, etc. I realised that personal relationships play a very important role in the health and growth of a business. Many times people don't work with you only for money. They do business with you even for a low margin because of your personal relationship.*
- *I was deeply influenced by KVS' habit of reading. He made me realise how much of his own wisdom is through the books he read. Encouraged by him, reading helped me In my thirties, to accumulate knowledge that other people gain much later in life.*

Nayan Bhai bid Kishore farewell with a glowing testament:

Kishore Bhai's whatever-it-takes attitude always works. More than the effort, it is this attitude that brought us success. I have learned a lot from him ... he has taught us this not by telling us ... but by living it.

The following are some of the important values that shaped me, and became part of Mangal's DNA.

- *Trust the people you work with*
- *Honesty is the foundation of any organization*
- *Have empathy for all and look for win-win solutions*
- *Being compassionate is important in a good leader*
- *Be collaborative*

While hiring staff, first look for their work ethic and their values. There are a lot of smart people, but good and smart people are few. Smartness without fundamental values is no good in the long run.

Being in procurement, his three beliefs helped us be the first to make Jacquard tablecloths and kitchen towels for the US market.

- *Knowledge is power*
- *Success is in the details*
- *Whatever it takes*

He had a habit of accounting for the details. He worked very hard and diligently to understand everything involved in production. Once he obtained the manufacturing knowledge of the required raw materials, machinery and entire production process, he was not only able to negotiate the best prices, but work collaboratively with the factory owners, managers or workers to get quality goods on a timely basis. Getting huge quantities for Walmart orders would not have been possible without this fine working style of KVS.

Kudos to Kishore Bhai! He was almost thirty years older than us, but with his meditation and passion for work, his energies were far greater than ours.

12

JOB INTERVIEW AT SEVENTY-ONE

It is the supreme art of the teacher to awaken joy in creative expression and knowledge.

—Albert Einstein

When Kishore moved to Coimbatore in 1990 by himself, he strove to build a social circle in the predominantly conservative city. Kishore never missed an opportunity to interact with strangers, whether it was on a bus ride to Chennapatnam or on a flight to Mumbai.

Among the earliest friends he made in Coimbatore were the couples, Jagadish and Renuka Bhojani and Krishnakumar and Jyoti Jobanputra. Kishore once mentioned to Jagadish Bhai that he now had his brother and two sisters in Coimbatore.

Along with two other families, that of Rajnikant and Lata Karia and Mukund and Sarla Suchde, the Jobanputras and the Sonpals formed a unique quartet of close friends. They would get together on Sundays, organizing potluck lunches of the choicest Gujarati savouries. In the otherwise conservative city, later Lata too looked forward to meeting this set of friends regularly.

In addition, Kishore joined the Rotary club. The talks were held mostly in Tamil and Kishore had a tough time following. However, he enjoyed networking over dinner subsequently and made a lot of friends. The club also conducted philanthropic activities like feeding the poor or visiting old age homes.

Early in 2009, during one such visit to an old age home, Kishore was offered a ride home by a fellow Rotarian, Mr Alagiriswamy, a practicing chartered accountant. The hour-long drive turned out to be highly engaging, as they discussed their background and experiences. They were both deeply influenced by Swami Vivekananda. Alagiriswamy was engaged with a few schools in the city. Ascertaining Kishore's vast experience and deep interest in pedagogy, Alagiriswamy invited Kishore for a speech at the annual day function of one of the schools, Geethanjalee Matric Higher Secondary School.

Over two hundred students were impressed by Kishore's speech and gave him a standing ovation. The experiences shared by Kishore were a source of learning and impressed Alagiriswamy. As a way of remembrance, Kishore gave out mementos to all the children. They all were touched by this gesture.

In February of that year, Alagiriswamy spoke to Kishore about a school where he was the treasurer. The school was looking for a senior person to be the registrar and enquired if Kishore was willing to consider the position. Kishore agreed and an informal meeting was set up with the chairman of the school, Dr B.K. Krishnaraj Vanavrayar.

The Chairman lived in Rukmini Nagar, a posh area in Coimbatore. As the conversation was to have been casual, Kishore was surprised on being treated rather formally, like it was an interview! He was asked about his background and past experience. When Kishore mentioned about his adulation for Ramakrishna Paramahamsa and Swami Vivekananda, the discussion changed track and became friendly. The Chairman was impressed to know that Kishore had visited the famous Belur Math way back in the 1960s. Kishore's eyes lit up when the Chairman mentioned the name of the school, Bharatiya Vidya Bhavan. The neighbourhood in which Kishore grew up as a child in Bombay also had a Bharatiya Vidya Bhavan, and Kishore had even met the founder of the mission long back.

The Chairman offered Kishore the position, where he would have to manage two schools as a registrar. Kishore was not familiar with the responsibilities of a Registrar, but he had always wanted to be involved in education so gladly accepted the offer.

When Kishore enquired about the joining date, he was surprised to hear the reply: '*The next day!*'

Finally, it was agreed upon that he would join in March, right after Holi. It was a surreal moment for Kishore when he, at age 71, received the appointment letter from the Chairman. On 12 March 2009, Kishore formally joined as the Registrar of Bharatiya Vidya Bhavan in Coimbatore. He was introduced to all the staff including the secretary, who was to familiarize Kishore with the functioning of the school and his role.

One of the two schools, located in the outskirts was still under construction. Kishore immediately involved himself in overseeing the construction, reminiscing his experiences of building the Permali house and his own bungalow in Bhopal.

After Kishore left Mangal, he missed the company of two people who were his pillars of strength during the stint—Anita, his office assistant and Sundaram, his faithful and trusted driver who was with him for fifteen years. Anita was his backbone, the secret behind Kishore's efficient work ethic despite his hectic schedule and frequent travel. Over time, she became more like family and Kishore even supported her daughter's education and wedding expenses, long after she had moved on and settled in her native, Kerala. Post Mangal, Sundaram decided to start his own trucking business, but stayed in touch with Kishore. Kishore's weekday schedule in the new role was quite different. He worked from nine in the morning till early afternoon, even on Saturdays. Right from reviewing expenses, overseeing salaries, looking through hiring, maintenance and procurement functions of the school, Kishore had a lot to manage, but within a couple of months, he was totally hands on and ready for more.

In the fortnightly review meeting, the Chairman was apprised of the pressing issue of providing an increment to the teachers, which had led to dissenting voices within the staff. Realizing that the finance head needed support, he requested Kishore to help. In his methodical and planned manner, Kishore conducted a thorough review of the budget, went through the balance sheet of the school in detail and made a clear list of options to address the teachers' grievances and came up with an amicable solution on the matter. The Chairman was impressed by the report and acknowledged that even experienced managers with an MBA degree would not have done such a diligent job.

The school had a busy calendar, full of academic and social activities, including music, dance, debate, drama and even lectures by eminent personalities. Kishore was a regular attendee to these events, and he would often enthrall the audience with motivational speeches.

It was during these events that Lata grew acquainted with the school, and was even called to care for students, especially the primary section, when teachers were on leave. Lata's accommodating and spontaneous offer to be involved in the school activities surprised Kishore. Only later did he realize this was also to ensure that he took care of his health and got back home in time for Lunch! She was fondly known as '*Patti*', grandmother in Tamil, among the younger kids in the school.

By June 2009, Kishore felt settled in his new role. One day, he received a surprise email from Hetal, inviting them for a vacation to Europe. While Kishore and Lata had made trips to the US and Japan to be with their children, they had not had a chance to travel to Europe. Hetal had made a travel plan for three weeks! Kishore was hesitant to ask for a leave, but the Chairman encouraged him to go for it and even suggested that he visit Bharatiya Vidya Bhavan in London as well.

That very evening, when Kishore reached home, Lata immediately asked him to be in front of the laptop. Their granddaughter, Hetal's child, Anusha, was on a video call. The moment he saw Anusha, Kishore was beaming. A wide smile spread across his face as Anusha described her day in school to them.

Kishore had always been fond of children. Right from taking care of his young sisters to his own children, Kishore was the source of knowledge, inspiration and even entertainment for all of them. With the advent of technology, physical meetings had reduced and virtual conversations increased, but that had not dampened Kishore's spirit and enthusiasm.

Right from carrying his three-year-old sister Jyoti around as she learnt to walk, to braiding four-year-old Renuka's hair, to scrubbing besan when giving bath to Manali, Kishore had done it all with ease. He played on swings and rode bikes with them, taught carrom, cards and chess to Anusha and discussed mythology with Manali's children, Aashka and Ayush. Kishore was not only comfortable, but also enjoyed the time with kids. He made an effort to have fun with them.

At Manali's house in Detroit, he spent hours in Barnes and Noble or the public library, reading children's book to later narrate them to the children, entertaining Aashka and Ayush with new information.

While at Hetal's house in Tokyo, he loved commuting by the public transport, the metro and buses, observing the Japanese and their style of living. He would then talk to Anusha about the things he had observed and what she could learn from these experiences. He taught and regularly played the card game Bridge with Hetal and Manali, when they were young and he continued the tradition by playing the card game *Bluff* with Anusha.

For Kishore, spending time with his grandchildren was not just about having fun. He looked at ways for them to learn from his experience. On one of the trips to Detroit, in an informal chat with Ayush, Kishore asked him, 'When do you cut your nails?'

'When they grow long,' replied Ayush.

Kishore smiled, as that was the answer he had expected. He said, 'No, you should have a fixed date/time in the week do it. Then it becomes a habit.'

Ayush was awestruck by the simplicity and the effectiveness of this advice and remembered it, whenever he found it hard to be regular at something.

Whether it was discussing technology with Hetal or hashing out details about the automotive industry with Apurva, his son-in-law who worked at General Motors, Kishore would do his research and read up relevant information to ensure a meaningful conversation. He would cite specific nuances of these industries and surprise even Hetal and Apurva.

In November 2009, the new school in the outskirts of Coimbatore was nearing completion, and the trust decided to set up a large statue of Lord Ganesh in the school, after conducting a Prana Prathista ceremony. Kishore had grown up in Bombay, and had often participated in the nine-day long Ganesh festival in the city. He was thus asked to lead the ceremony and the prayer. Despite the unexpected heavy rains that lashed the city on that day, Kishore left home at 4:15 a.m.

to reach school at sharp 5 a.m. for the ceremony. The Chairman was touched by the level of sincerity that Kishore displayed in every activity.

Through his vast knowledge, affectionate, humble and giving nature, Kishore became very popular at the school, among students and staff alike. On the 150th birth anniversary of Swami Vivekananda, Kishore lead the school celebrations in his honour. They set up posters of Swamiji, donated books, and set up a Vivekananda Study centre.

Over a period of time, the Chairman also observed that the spirit of discipline and diligence that Kishore emphasized on, had trickled down and spread among the staff, leading to an invigorating atmosphere in the school. Apart from the official meetings in the school, Kishore often had many long discussions with the Chairman. During one of these informal chats, Kishore shared his interest in reading biographies of leaders like Jawaharlal Nehru, Mahatma Gandhi, Vinoba Bhave. The Chairman and Kishore would subsequently exchange books on a regular basis. Kishore presented one of his favourite books to him, titled *Inspirational Gems.* Kishore had kept up the habit of lending/gifting books to others, and he had in fact, distributed hundred copies of this book. The family physician and a close friend, attributes his friendship with Kishore to the book he received as a gift on their very first meeting. Impressed by Kishore's ardent love for Vinoba Bhave, the Chairman made a portrait of Acharya ji and gave it to Kishore as a surprise gift.

Kishore also attended many social functions as a representative of the school and soon became quite popular in Coimbatore. Despite knowing very little Tamil, he was able to build a strong rapport with everyone. Kishore earned a lot of respect and admiration.

At the Rotary Club, Kishore soon became a well-known senior member of Coimbatore West branch. He was also very active in the local Gujarati community through the Gujarati

Samaj. Lata and Kishore regularly attended meetings and kept in touch with the members. Kishore amused his friends and acquaintances by minutely recalling details about their interactions. Lata, not one to be left behind, was quite active in the sister wing of Rotary, Innerwheel. Not only would she regularly attend the meetings, but also participate in various fun events, food donation drives and other charity activities.

One day in August 2013, Kishore was surprised by a phone call.

'Pappa, we are coming to Coimbatore next weekend,' Hetal said. He was then based in Gurgaon, and planned to come with his family.

'What's the occasion? Are all of you coming?' Kishore was pleasantly surprised.

'Occasion? It's your birthday Pappa!'

Kishore smiled. 'Of course, I know. I may be getting old, but I haven't forgotten my own birthday.'

'Pappa, but it's not just any other birthday. You are turning 75! And we want to have a big party to celebrate the milestone,' Hetal said, surprising Kishore further. Hetal had already discussed this with his mother, and they all were excited. They just had to get Kishore, the man of the party, onboard with the plan.

'A party? I have never had a birthday party in my life; why have one at 75?'

'All the more reason to do it, Pappa. It's your platinum jubilee.' Kishore loved celebrations, but he had never thrown a party, so he reluctantly agreed. They realized that it would inconvenience many to travel from Bombay and Gujarat, so Kishore suggested they have two separate celebrations— a party at the Cosmopolitan Club in Coimbatore, and a Gayatri Havan (fire ritual) in Lonawala, a place short drive from Bombay.

Both of these events were grand. Pravin and his wife, Jyoti flew down from Bombay, as did Kishore's sisters from Chennai, and all his old and new colleagues and friends, business partners from all across Tamil Nadu graced the occasion on 21 August 2013. Amidst them all, Kishore felt humbled and nostalgic as he traced back the eventful seventy-five years of life. He had survived a tough childhood, and faced struggles and triumphs in his personal life and career—he had indeed come far. He had come out stronger, more knowledgeable and was grateful to have his near and dear ones grace the solemn occasion.

Subsequently, the year 2019 started off on a high note for Kishore. The school planned a grand celebration for the 150th birth anniversary of Mahatma Gandhi. On 2 January, the school was to host a special guest, Ela Gandhi, granddaughter of Mahatma Gandhi. Kishore ensured the success of this event and felt great to be part of it, reminiscing all the old memories he had of Gandhiji, right from the days of India's freedom struggle. Among the attendees were noted historian, Ramachandra Guha and Kezevino Aram, president of the Shanti Ashram.

As the decade came to a close, Kishore continued to organize the school's activities, reviewing the budget and streamlining the finances. His role grew more and more pivotal in the daily functioning of the school, as Kishore grew older.

In January 2020, even though his health was faltering, Kishore and Lata made a trip to Mumbai to attend a couple of family weddings. Apart from meeting close friends and family, they also witnessed Hetal running his third Mumbai Marathon. Subsequently, they drove down to Pune and Kishore had a small rendezvous with Krishnakumar and Pravin and the three friends had a great time reminiscing their good old school days.

Kishore, through his hard work, dedication and resilience left a big mark on Bharatiya Vidya Bhavan. He remained true to the pledge he had taken: *he would work there until his last breath.* He served actively till 10 March 2020, when his health finally failed him. Kishore applied for a short leave, but it ended up being far longer than he had planned.

In words of Mr Alagiriswamy, the Treasurer at Bharatiya Vidya Bhavan:

We are what we repeatedly do; excellence, then, is not an act but a habit.

—Aristotle

A great example of the above was Mr Sonpal, a man of excellence. Mr Sonpal had once quoted Swami Vivekananda, stating: 'We have to be silent and take the journey inwards when our soul is the best teacher for spiritual growth.' Only a man like Mr Sonpal, can actually live through and demonstrate the learning of someone like Swami Vivekananda.

13

THE BIG FIGHT

Here is the test to find whether your mission on earth is finished: If you're alive, it isn't.

—Richard Bach

Hetal turned in his sleep and noticed the light was on in the bathroom. The bedside clock indicated: 00:58; he had two minutes. He immediately sprang into action.

Sorbi tablet? Check
Volini lotion? Check
Hingwati tablets? Check
Chinese Balm? Check
Windows open? Check
Mosquito net opened? Check

Every night, precisely at 1 a.m., Kishore would use the washroom. The moments right after he came out of the washroom were very painful for him. He would immediately lie down, and have a seizure that left him breathless.

Kishore trudged out of the bathroom and lay down on the bed. Within seconds he was shouting in pain, 'Open the window, fast! Remove the mosquito net, I cannot breathe!' As Hetal comforted him, he looked towards the fan. 'Increase the speed, I cannot breathe.'

'Oops!' Hetal exclaimed as he leapt to reach out for the regulator.

'Lata!' Kishore called out.

Lata entered as Hetal started massaging his legs with the prescribed oil. Light flooded the room. Lata's weak eyesight meant she had poor vision in the night, but she was familiar with the process. She rushed to Kishore's side. Hetal passed the bottle of Chinese balm across to her, so she could apply it on Kishore's chest. Kishore kept instructing both of them through the pain.

Kishore had only relaxed for a moment.

'Close the window, I told you to close it,' Kishore screamed.

Hetal noticed Kishore was shivering. His body shook from head to toe in pain. His eyes were clouded with fear. Hetal dropped the Volini tube from his hand as he quickly shut the window with a loud thud. On any other day, Hetal would have worried that the noise would disturb the neighbours. Tonight, he was only worried about his father.

'*Madame, hu jawano chu* (Madam, I think I am dying),' Kishore looked up at Lata, his eyes moist.

Hetal was taken aback for a moment. His father had faced countless hardships in life, but he had never seen him acknowledge any pain. While growing up, Hetal never saw his father sick, even for a day. By his own admission, throughout the eighty years of his life, this was only the third time that his father had fallen 'sick.'

Realizing that there was no point holding back the strong

medication, Hetal grabbed the strip of Sorbi tablet and took out one and placed it under Kishore's tongue. A few seconds later, Kishore's breathing began to ease.

Hetal looked at the wall clock: 01:13. The last few minutes had seemed like the toughest fifteen minutes of his life. By the time Lata returned with a glass of water, Kishore's eyes were closed and he was fast asleep. Hetal gently pulled over the blanket for him and switched off the lights. The next attack would happen at 4 a.m.

It was 7 a.m. when Hetal finally woke up. He turned to his right and saw his father sleeping peacefully; there were no signs of the pain he had gone through in the night. He would wake up in a few hours and have his morning tea and breakfast without any more trouble.

The problem had started a few weeks back, in February 2019. Lata had called Hetal to inform that Kishore's appetite had decreased. He looked frail and lethargic, and she mentioned that he slept through most of the day. While he insisted on going to work, to Bharatiya Vidya Bhavan, he clearly lacked the enthusiasm he had earlier. Hetal was in Gurgaon and was not sure what to make of the situation. He immediately called Manali in Detroit and gave her an update. She recommended that they get a blood test done for Kishore.

Kishore was averse to allopathic medicine, much like his own father before him. So Hetal devised a plan. He called and told him that he had received a coupon for a free health check-up and wanted him to avail it. '*Oh, free ma chey*?' (It is free?) he asked.

'Yes Pappa, it is, and they will come home to collect the sample,' Hetal assured him.

When Hetal got the test report on email the next day, he immediately forwarded it to their family physician in Coimbatore. They had known Dr Raju for over twenty years. On assessing the low platelet count, doctor recommended that

PSA test be done immediately.

The test confirmed Dr Raju's worst fear. *His PSA was 1500,* as compared to normal level of 0-4. Dr Raju recommended they meet a urologist. When Hetal mentioned this to Kishore, he immediately recognized the name of the urologist.

'Oh, I know him. I had met him last year. My PSA was 49 then. He had asked me to get a biopsy done, but you know the condition of my heart,' he said.

Apparently, his cardiologist advised against the biopsy as his heart was not strong enough for the same.

Subsequently, Kishore had consulted a famous naturopath in Ahmedabad and the PSA had come down through the treatment, so he forgot about getting back to the urologist.

This time, the urologist recommended further tests, which revealed what was feared all along.

Kishore had last stage prostate cancer. Hetal had returned to Gurgaon, and was shocked to get the email. He read the report, trying to decipher the technical terms amidst all the high-resolution images of his father's body. He shared the report with Dr Raju on email and then called him. He had gone through the report and suggested that Kishore be provided palliative treatment. The term was new to Hetal and he assumed it must be some form of cure. However, his jaw dropped when he saw the meaning online: '*Care for the Terminally ill*'. Hetal could not believe it, 'No, I am not going to let cancer take my father away'. He swore to himself.

They were subsequently recommended to meet the oncologist, Dr Sudhakar at the Royal Care Hospital. They decided to meet Kishore's cardiologist prior to the meeting with the oncologist. The cardiologist glanced through the reports, and then gazed at them questioningly. He indicated to the nurse to help Kishore be wheeled out, so they could talk in private.

'Let's see, he has to fight this cancer, his lungs are weak

due to tuberculosis earlier and his heart blockages makes it even more complicated.'

Hetal sat astounded. He knew nothing about his father's heart blockages and apparently, neither did his mother.

'Mr Sonpal has had multiple heart blockages for more than twelve years now. First diagnosed in 2006, when he complained about breathing issues. Your father just refused any kind of surgical treatment and was prescribed a set of medicines.'

On seeing the puzzled expressions on their faces, the doctor understood that Kishore had kept this from the family.

'Look, he has proved himself right. If he can survive twelve years on oral tablets, he clearly did not need the surgery.'

'He is a strong man, I admire his courage,' he said as they left to visit the oncologist, hope rising in hearts of Kishore's family members.

Kishore looked positive after the first meeting with the oncologist, and felt that he had found his saviour in Dr Sudhakar. The doctor prescribed two tablets to be taken daily, apart from a couple of injections that were to be taken every three months. Chemotherapy was not advisable at this stage as Kishore was quite weak.

During the first two weeks of his treatment, Kishore showed good improvement. He became more energetic, his appetite had gone up and he was keen to get back to work. Lata and Hetal were glad to see his cheerful self again.

But by the third week, he again became lethargic and complained of back pain. The doctor recommended tests, and it was confirmed that the PSA had actually shot up. *It was 2603 now.* Indicating this was nothing but just a 'flare', the doctor advised that they wait for another two weeks before making any judgment regarding the treatment.

As a motivational speaker, Hetal had been giving lectures at many business schools in India. However, his dream was to give a talk with his father in the audience. So he approached the

Chairman for a talk at Bharatiya Vidya Bhavan. The Chairman gladly agreed to the proposal and the talk was scheduled for 29 July 2019.

A day prior to the event, Lata told Hetal that his father was not in a position to attend the talk at the school. Hetal was not ready to accept it. He went to Kishore's room to check on him. His father was on his favourite rocking chair, reading a book.

Kishore was excited to see his son, and said, 'I am sure the children are going to love your talk. What grades are you going to address?' he asked with a pained hug.

'Grades 11 and 12. I plan to talk about career planning,' Hetal replied

Kishore smiled and wished him luck. He put his book aside and was fast asleep within minutes. He really did not have enough strength to go to the school, Hetal realized.

The next morning was a strange one. Hetal dressed, got ready and had breakfast with Kishore as always. But instead of Kishore, it was his son who left for the school. Hetal however noticed no sign of disappointment on his father's face. He shook Hetal's hand and wished him luck. Hetal reminded his mother to video call him, so his father could at least watch him virtually.

On stage, Hetal referred to Kishore as his ideal and his biggest source of learning and inspiration. He encouraged students to break the shackles of expectations. His father was fine to not to expect to have the strength to attend *his son's* talk in *his* school; he had accepted it. The speech was exhilarating and Hetal received a thundering applause from auditorium full of students. But what mattered most to Hetal was to see his father's beaming face and moist eyes on the video call at the end of the talk. He had tears of joy.

'Start accepting!' Kishore said, his eyes glittering.

'I was waiting for you to say that!' Kishore said to Hetal as he returned home. Completing the quote that Kishore used to give as an advice all the time: 'Stop Expecting, Start Accepting.'

A month later, a week before Kishore's eighty-first birthday, he received the best birthday gift. Kishore's report showed that his PSA had come down drastically. Dr Sudhakar was quite surprised by the remarkable dip, and they were all overjoyed. But the problems had not ceased in entirety, as the PSA was still high; treatment was to be continued.

Later, Hetal candidly asked his father why he had ignored medical advice to get a biopsy. Kishore told him that in 2018, when he was diagnosed with TB and had had a rigorous eleven-month medication schedule, it had killed his appetite and made him weak. When the doctor mentioned the biopsy, Kishore had suspected cancer. He feared the complex cancer treatment and chemotherapy that he would have to go through.

The month of September brought improvement in Kishore. He gradually was back to his daily routine and resumed going to school too. He spent the mornings at Bharatiya Vidya Bhavan, and then rested in the afternoon. His appetite had become almost normal, ate a healthy dinner and went to sleep early every night. In the meanwhile, Lata's health had deteriorated but she put up a brave face for her husband, tirelessly managing everything.

However, on 2 October 2019, Lata had an unfortunate accident at a mall that evening. She was out shopping for Diwali, picking up sarees for all the maids. She slipped while stepping out of the elevator and fell on her back. As she fell backwards, she heard a cracking noise and sensed her back had given in. Fortunately, people in the elevator helped her to her car and the driver drove her straight to the nearby hospital. She was in excruciating pain. The x-ray confirmed that she had a fractured spine. She needed six weeks of bed rest.

The next day, the roles were reversed. Kishore, who often complained that he had to be alone at home while Lata stepped out for errands, was himself going out now, even shopping for vegetables at the market. Their love had always stood testament to a deep bond, and their sense of responsibility towards each other had never weakened. Lata had initially been afraid to inform Kishore about the accident, not sure how he would react. But two weeks later, she was amazed to see Kishore busy in the kitchen, cooking an entire meal for her!

In the month of October, Hetal travelled to Goa for a wedding in the family. During the trip, he came across a naturopath, Dr Anysia; she had miraculously cured his meniscus tear in the left knee. She mentioned about having cured cancer in some of her patients as well. Hetal invited her to Coimbatore during Diwali break and see his father, and she gladly agreed.

On Diwali day in 2019 at home in Coimbatore, Dr Anysia treated Kishore with the cupping therapy of healing and prescribed some medicines and natural supplements. She emphasized that oxygen had to be taken regularly. Kishore agreed to diligently follow the routine. Ironically, while Kishore had hoped to replace his box of allopathic medicines with naturopathic ones, many new tablets just got added to his regimen instead. He remarked that he felt like he was consuming more medicines than food!

They were in for another pleasant surprise after the next PSA test, three weeks into the naturopathic treatment. The PSA had come down to just nine! It was still double of normal but much lower than before.

When they met Dr Sudhakar with the report, his response was guarded. He was pleased about Kishore's progress, but wanted to wait for a month and observe him further. Kishore's willpower and positivity had surprised him.

Later, Kishore mentioned that he received positive vibes from the doctor's cabin, that it had the feel of a temple, which gave him confidence.

The months of November and December flew by, as Kishore had many visitors from out of town. His sisters, Jyoti and Renuka, stayed over for a couple of weeks, making him his favourite meals. Lata too was glad to have the additional help and support. She was seventy-six years old and had her own health issues. Hiten Bhai, along with his wife, Neeta, also visited from Mumbai. Over the course of elaborate meals and detailed discussions, reminiscent of the 'Swadhyay' sessions they used to have earlier, they talked about the times they had during the Mangal journey. Manali came over from Detroit and spent two memorable weeks with them.

The next blood test was due for mid-December. Anxiety ran high. While Kishore had been taking medicines regularly, he continued to work at school and the daily chores took a toll on his health. Of course, he would not admit feeling weak and maintained his calm demeanour, even when confronted by the doctor.

Dr Sudhakar had a wide smile on his face when he received a copy of the next blood test. Good news! The PSA had remained stable. Kishore had proved his detractors wrong, including the doctor who had signed off on him and had advocated palliative care. Once again in life, through sheer willpower, dedication and unflinching faith in God, Kishore had pulled off the virtually impossible. He had fought cancer and emerged on the other side with a triumphant smile.

14

THE GREEN MILE

I know God will not give me anything I can't handle. I just wish He didn't trust me so much.

—Mother Teresa

'Pappa, I will arrive a day before you and Mummy,' Hetal said on the phone. Hetal had already received his father's itinerary.

'Oh, you plan to be in Mumbai on Saturday. You can come to pick us up at the airport. But why are you coming earlier? We haven't booked a room for Saturday. Should I call them?' Even at eighty-one, Kishore was still worried about his son, the forty-five-year-old Hetal, as if he were still a child.

'Don't worry. I'll stay with Masi (Aunt) in Walkeshwar,' Hetal assured him. 'I will be running the Mumbai Marathon on Saturday morning. I should be done by 10 a.m., if not earlier. I will have enough time to see you at the airport.' Hetal replied.

Kishore wished him good luck.

On 19 January 2020 at about 8:30 a.m. as Hetal was running the stretch on Worli sea face, with the NSCI grounds to his left and the Arabian Sea shimmering on his right; he could see the bright Haji Ali ahead. Earlier in the morning, he had decided to dedicate the medal he would receive for running the marathon to his mother. She had been a silent force throughout his life, tirelessly working behind the scenes, holding the fort—whether in Bhopal or Coimbatore—diligently taking care of Manali and himself while their father was busy fighting his numerous battles.

However, once he had finished the marathon he realized that the Tata Mumbai Marathon awards not one, but two medals to all the finishers. The second medal is for the runner's coach. This worked out well for Hetal; his father, his lifelong coach, deserved to get the other medal.

Hetal met his parents outside the Mumbai airport as the airline staff wheeled them out. With a flourish, he presented them with the two medals. He thanked both of them profusely, reminding them how they both had been his pillars of strength in his life. Neither of them had ever received a medal before and they were touched by this gesture.

Kishore and Lata were in Mumbai to attend the wedding of Dhiren's daughter, Esha. Kishore was also keen to meet his numerous friends and relatives in the city. He sensed that time was not on his side and he wanted to make the most of this opportunity. He was very fortunate that not only were they able to meet all of their family members, they could also travel to Pune and meet Kishore's childhood friends, Krishnakumar and Pravin.

A day before their return to Coimbatore, after having spent fourteen days in Mumbai, Hetal called his father. Kishore sounded weak and it seemed that the trip had taken a toll on him. Hetal immediately spoke to Dr Sudhakar and he suggested a few routine tests be done immediately after they return to Coimbatore.

The test results on 14 February 2020 were not very encouraging; the PSA had gone up to ninety-nine. The doctor increased the medicine dosage and hoped for the best.

After they returned from Mumbai, Kishore resumed work at the school. Lata was concerned about his health, but Kishore would not listen. So, she tried a different option. She called Hetal in Gurgaon and asked *him* to convince his father to spend less time at the school. When that too failed, Lata called the Chairman. Kishore was ordered to leave; he went home immediately, and ate well and then rested.

By this time, Kishore was used to the dietary restrictions that he had to follow. But he was a foodie at heart and craved for the very things that were prohibited. Sweets, salty snacks, fried stuff: he was missing it all. Right from childhood, Kishore had a weakness for Gujarati sweets. His sisters often made his favourite Indian sweets and would courier them to him. Lata would be exasperated by the amount of ghee and sugar in the sweets and her first instinct was to hide them. But Kishore's strong sense of smell would foil such plans and he would demand the sweets. During a routine visit to the doctor, Kishore decided to seek the doctor's help for a permanent fix.

Dr Sudhadar laughed and gave him permission, 'Not just sweets, it's okay for him to even have ice cream.' Kishore was overjoyed and called Lata on the drive back home, 'Please make sure Radha (the house maid) makes *Sheero* (a sweet item) for me. That will be my lunch today!'

His mobility had been limited by the illness, but Kishore worked out ingenious ways to conserve his energy—walking in short bursts from the bedroom to the living room. Here he would sit on his favourite rocking chair and watch television or read. Though the cancer had taken a toll on his physical health, his mind was as sharp as ever. His sense of smell was strong, and sitting in bedroom, he knew when food was cooked and when the gas needed to be switched off. He would read a lot, often picking up some of his favourite books to re-read. His memory was still very strong.

Hetal would visit them often and on little pretext. On one such trip, Hetal landed in Coimbatore on Saturday, 8th of March 2020, in the morning, as he decided to have breakfast with his father. On the way from the airport, he picked up idlis from People's Park, Kishore's favourite South Indian joint and they had a sumptuous breakfast at home. Next day evening, Hetal returned back to Gurgaon.

The very next day Kishore and Lata attended the seventieth birthday celebration of Jyoti Jubanputra, their family friend. The subsequent morning, at about 7:30 a.m. when Hetal called home Kishore apologized for not being able to call earlier.

'We woke up late,' he said, 'and Mummy has some problem in her eye.'

Hetal was surprised by his father's tone, 'What kind of problem?' he asked.

'Mummy's right eye is black and swollen. She cannot open it,' Kishore explained.

Hetal immediately switched to a video call. Lata tried to downplay the injury so that her son would not worry. But she had not realized she was on video and Hetal could see her face. Hetal convinced her to see a doctor immediately. He requested their next-door neighbour, Vikashni to take his mother to the hospital. In the afternoon, Vikashni called to let Hetal know that everything was fine. The eye doctor had prescribed a balm and some medicines.

Hetal was not convinced so he took the late afternoon flight to Coimbatore. When he reached home in the evening, the black swelling below Lata's eye had increased, and she also complained of a mild headache.

The next day, the black bruise had spread even further and

now looked scary. It covered the entire left side of her face. They went to the general physician in the hospital, as it was not just an eye problem. There they learnt that the bump could be attributed to a possible fall, but Lata could not recollect any such event. She did notice some vomit on her bed and clothes, but did not think she had fallen down. Considering her weakness and low platelet count, the doctor advised that they admit her immediately to the hospital.

Lata's stay at the hospital was quite challenging for the family. When Hetal told Kishore about it, he wanted to visit her at the hospital. But he was quite weak himself and it was not advisable. The COVID-19 cases were increasing in the country and lot of precautions were advised for the elderly. Hetal would be with Lata at the hospital till breakfast, and then come home to prepare breakfast for Kishore. He would subsequently go back and forth between home and the hospital, ensuring he would give company to both parents for each meal.

After three days in the hospital, with the platelet count improving marginally, Lata had regained her strength and they could convince the doctor to discharge her. When she returned home she immediately took charge of all the tasks at home. Despite Hetal's protests, she was keen to get back to her normal routine at the earliest.

In the subsequent week, when they met Dr Sudhakar for Kishore's monthly injection and tests, there was a cause for concern. His PSA had gone up again. Another drug was prescribed, but this one was known to have side effects: muscle soreness, joint pain, headaches, and backache.

Within a week of taking the new tablets, they observed some of the expected side effects. Kishore complained of back pain, and needed an ice-pack on his back to feel comfortable. Lata and Hetal took turns massaging his head and aching legs. His appetite too had gone down, leading to more weakness.

In the meantime, the Corona virus cases in the country

were rising rapidly, and the pandemic had spread. Prime Minister Modi announced a nation-wide lockdown for three weeks. This proved to be a blessing in disguise as Hetal could continue to stay with his parents and work from home. But Kishore struggled to adjust with the home isolation rules of the pandemic. He did not like that neither could he leave his apartment to visit the school, nor could anyone come to meet him.

More than the lockdown-induced challenges; Kishore had his own battles to fight. The PSA test in mid-April brought more bad news. The cancer cells had increased and the doctor indicated that the new medication would have to continue.

May brought some relief after the lockdown norms were relaxed a bit. But Hetal continued his stay in Coimbatore, as flights were still not operational. With the migrant labour crisis impacting testing lab staff, he had to take his father to the hospital even for the blood-test, as home collection of sample was not possible. Kishore now had to be taken on a wheelchair, as he was too weak to walk much.

'Please be ready by 10 a.m. tomorrow,' Hetal told Kishore the previous evening, reminding him of the doctor's appointment the next day. In the morning, Kishore was so weak that even taking a shower required a lot of effort.

'I need to lie down for five minutes, then we can leave,' Kishore told Hetal as he walked into his room at 9:50 the next day morning. Hetal was surprised to see Kishore had shaved and showered all by himself. But he was in visible pain.

Despite the pain and discomfort, his brain was as sharp as ever. He had promised Dr Sudhakar a few books in the previous meeting, and he reminded Hetal to take them along.

The meeting with Dr Sudhakar on 20 May was crucial. They had a tough decision to make. They could start a new mediation or opt for chemotherapy. The topic was discussed in detail on the phone with Manali and Khyati as well, who, after completing her PhD, was now working with Pfizer and was well-versed in cancer treatment. Kishore preferred medication with fewer side effects and hence they went for an oral tablet and injection, choosing not to go with chemotherapy.

A week after the meeting with the doctor, on 27 May, they celebrated Hetal's forty-sixth birthday, his first in Coimbatore with his parents. It had been thirty years since he had spent so much time with his parents.

During the first week of June, the home isolation norms were relaxed and it was possible for them to have visitors. Mr Chandrashekar, business partner from Kishore's Mangal days, came down from Chennimalai to spend an evening with Kishore. Subsequently, Jyoti Jobanputra and her son, Mihir, also visited him. Incidentally, Krishnakumar Jobanputra had passed away in 2016, after a long and valiant battle with cancer.

By this time, Kishore had become very weak and was bed-ridden most of the time. On 11 June in the morning, his weakness had increased even further and he could not sit up without support. His blood sample had been collected the previous day and they requested a doctor to visit them at home. The doctor observed the low sodium level in the blood report and immediately recommended that Kishore be admitted to the hospital. He could be administered the right medication and be constantly monitored there. However, Kishore disliked going to hospital and the virus scare was another reason to dissuade the family from admitting him there.

The doctor assured Hetal that COVID-19 cases were handled in a separate section, and that his father would not come into contact with anyone dealing with the corona patients. Finally, they agreed to get Kishore admitted to the hospital. When the ambulance arrived later, Kishore refused to leave on a stretcher and insisted they get him a wheelchair. Fortunately one was available in the apartment itself.

While it took a long time to complete the admission process, the doctor visited him soon after and explained the treatment to the nurse on duty. Kishore was settled into a private room and given oxygen through a tube going into his nose. He had a sodium and IV drip administered as well. The ordeal was extremely painful for Kishore, who was very uncomfortable on the air mattress that had been provided. He commented that he felt like a caged tiger, despite the best efforts of the nurses and the doctors to make him comfortable.

After Lata went home in the evening, it was a struggle for the nurses to feed Kishore his dinner, a plain meal of ragi soup. The extra dose of medicines, the constant discomfort of all the tubes and an alien environment were in complete contrast to the safe confines of his home. It greatly frustrated Kishore, and it took the nurses almost an hour to feed him.

At 10.45 p.m., after the nurses had left the room and the lights had been dimmed, Kishore asked Hetal about Lata. Hetal told him that she was fine.

'She's had her dinner and was planning to sleep soon,' Hetal told his father.

'She has had her dinner and is sleeping? That's good.' Kishore replied and momentarily closed his eyes.

As Hetal lay down on the adjoining bed, he reflected on what a long day it had been. Next to him, Kishore was mumbling incoherently. Hetal gently asked him to try to rest and get some sleep. Hetal observed him till 11.45 p.m., when his father finally stopped mumbling, closed his eyes and turned to his right. Assured that his father was finally getting some rest, Hetal too shut his eyes and soon was fast asleep.

Hetal suddenly woke up and noticed lot of commotion in the room and that the lights were switched on by the nurse. The meter next to Kishore's bed displayed a low signal, and the nurse immediately called for the doctor on duty. Hetal rose from the bed, totally dazed and tried to make sense of what was going on. It was about 1 a.m. in the night, less than an hour since they had gone to sleep.

Kishore lay motionless on his bed.

Hetal stood next to him, dumbfounded. The doctor gently requested Hetal to step out of the room. They would attempt to resuscitate his father. Hetal dragged himself out of the room, hating the fact that he could do nothing for his father at that moment.

At 1:24 a.m., the doctor came out of the room and conveyed the news:

Kishore Vinodrai Sonpal, the small boy from Ahmedabad, who rose to become an engineer, went on to create a legacy for himself and brought joy to hundreds of people, after an eventful life of eighty-one years and 296 days, had left for his last journey to heaven.

AUTHOR'S NOTE

This book has been my life's most important project. Others earlier had approached Pappa to write his biography and he had not thought about it seriously. But when I proposed the plan to him, he immediately agreed to it. The experience of going through his life's journey has taught me a lot and I hope that the book will be a source of learning for many others.

A couple of years ago, I was moved and inspired by Mitch Albom's book, *Tuesdays with Morrie*. I too lived Mitch's life as I wrote the book. I would travel from Gurgaon to Coimbatore, spend weekends to hear Pappa share his stories, his life learnings and take notes. I feel great that I can share with the world, all that my father did and what he taught me.

Pappa had earlier chanced upon a fabulous book, *Die Empty* written by Todd Henry and he discussed it with me. He was moved by the concept. And true to what the book says, he did not die empty. He ensured that all knowledge and his life learning did not go away with him. His voice echoes throughout this book. It contains the details of his life: his conversations, all that he shared with me, without any modifications, straight from the heart.

Since his cancer was in the last stage, Pappa knew he would not survive long. He wanted to know what people thought about him *while he was alive.* He wanted feedback on his life. He received commendations from many of his friends, colleagues and family, and it was these commendations that kept him going as life got more and more challenging in his last few months. The notes took Pappa back to the times he spent with all of them. It gave him hope to stay strong and carry on living. The gratitude, love and affection showered by everyone gave him a sense of comfort and satisfaction that his time on this planet, had been well spent.

When I look back on how his life transpired, right from his childhood to the fifty plus years of professional life, I am amazed by the numerous challenges he overcame. He not only supported himself and his family, but also helped many others along the way. He was witness to major developments in India's history—right from the freedom struggle lead by Mahatma Gandhi, the wars India had with its neighbouring countries, India's industrial growth post-independence and the subsequent end of Licence Raj to ensuing liberalisation, the technology revolution in the new millennium and finally the CoVid pandemic.

Even at the age of seventy-one, when he could have happily retired from active life, he gave his life a new meaning by dedicating himself to Bharatiya Vidya Bhavan and giving back to the student community.

We were overwhelmed by the condolence messages that poured in on his death; so many people shared stories of how Pappa helped and influenced them. Pappa was the purest soul I have ever come across, and I do not say that just as a son.

Concluding a book is as hard as beginning one. I hope I have captured everything, and not missed anything important. As an author, I am sure I will have opportunities to write more books. But there will never be another Kishore. Pure souls like him come once in a lifetime. I live on with his learning, his memories, his blessings and the immense love that he gave all of us, now and forever.

ACKNOWLEDGEMENTS

The hardest part of writing the acknowledgements is noting every single person that has contributed and shaped this book. I sincerely apologize in advance if I have missed thanking anyone here.

The deepest of gratitude and the very reason this book came to life is, of course, to my father, Kishore Sonpal. After his death, a few friends commented how unfortunate it was that he could not see the book published. But I told them that even without seeing the printed version, he knew the book and its story from within and that he had a lot of faith in me to write it well.

With the book, the world now knows about my father. But a story is yet untold—that of my mother, Lata Sonpal. She has worked tirelessly all through her life and has been a constant source of motivation and support for the whole family. Her contribution and constant encouragement helped me tremendously while working on this project.

There are many people without whose contribution this book would not have been completed. First and foremost, I need to thank my dearest daughter, Anusha, my nephew, Ayush and my niece, Aashka. Right after I proposed the idea to my father, these three teenagers helped me structure and plan this book: What the chapters should be what the format would be, what all to include, and so on. They created a Google doc to aid me in writing the drafts and even reviewed the first few chapters. My sister, Manali, too shared a lot of feedback on the content and structure of the book and provided constant support in my writing journey, right from day one.

Next, I wish to thank all the family members and my father's friends and colleagues who sent in their commendation and notes. All the notes were sincere and deeply heartwarming for my father to read. The inputs from all of you helped me while I was writing and I cannot thank you enough for what those notes meant to my father during the last few months of his life.

I would also like to thank my friends, Adarsh Vatal, Ravi Vyas, Ravi Trivedi, Rohit Bhalla, Pawan Raj Kumar, Shubhangi Kapoor, Seju Shah and Sukant Bhattacharjee for having read the early and final versions of the manuscript and providing valuable suggestions.

Special thanks to Tomichan Mathew sir, my English teacher from Campion school, who edited the initial version of the manuscript and patiently responded to me, chapter by chapter. Also thanks to my old friend Peyush Agarwal, who applied his design expertise and prepared a beautiful book cover.

I would especially like to thank Chairman Sir, Dr B.K. Krishnaraj Vanavarayar, for kindly agreeing to write the foreword for this book. I must also mention Amit Somani, Ramesh Emani and Rajesh Kalra for reviewing the manuscript and also providing a quote for the book you now hold in your hands.

Thanks to Sanil Sachar for having given crucial inputs in the initial stages and also introducing me to Kanishka Gupta who is a great agent to work with.

Thanks a ton to Dibakar Ghosh and the team at Rupa Publications who helped me at every step of the publishing process.

THE FAMILY TREE

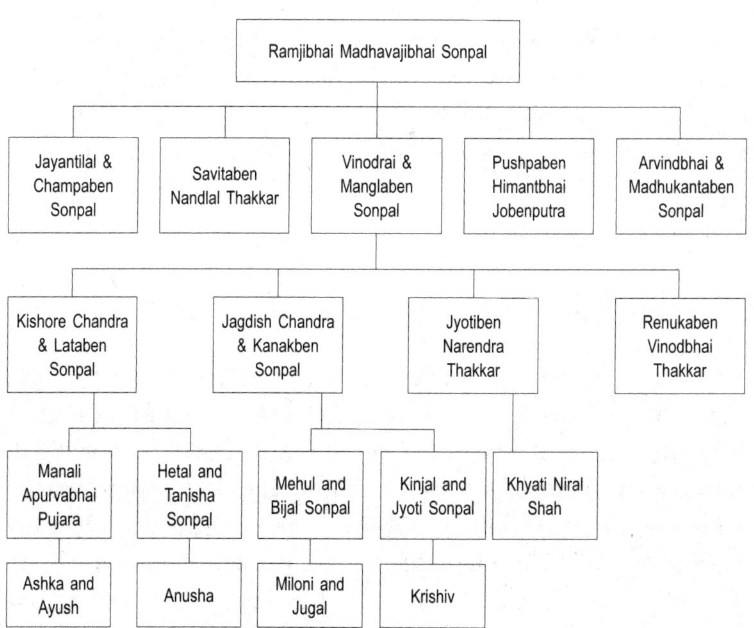

MUSINGS OF KISHORE

This section contains the articles, notes and diary entries that inspired Kishore V. Sonpal throughout his life. An avid reader and very regular at journaling, Kishore made it a point to write about all that had inspired him in his diaries. Here, I share the wealth—a collection of the best articles and quotes from his diaries.

FRUITS OF SELF CONTAINMENT

Every human being wants to be happy. Yet, in the real sense, very few have achieved happiness. Happiness is not a thing or a commodity that can be purchased in the market, nor it can be created artificially. One has to accept that happiness, for which one is struggling to acquire from the outside, is already within oneself. The mentality of the present generation is to watch for the door which is closed to open, but never to use the door which is already open. That is to say, man will not enjoy what he possesses but will waste his entire precious time trying to achieve what others have.

One will naturally be eager to know how to enjoy real happiness, which is within oneself. The first and very important thing that is required to become happy is to be simple. You can achieve everything if you are simple. Simplicity in life is the very first step to lift you to heavenly happiness.

If you are simple, you will not crave for things that are mundane and you will not feel jealousy towards those who possess more and better things than you. This will make you free from the madness of possessing things. Kindly keep in mind that happiness does not lie in possessing things but in enjoying what you have. A landlord may have ten buildings but he can enjoy only the house in which he lives. If you are simple, your requirements will be small as compared to others. Hence, you will not have to struggle endlessly to obtain things.

The second thought that comes to the mind is 'how to be simple'? By simplicity, I do not mean being simple merely in matters of dress, food, etc. Simplicity should pervade each and every sphere of human activity. This can be obtained only if you have contentment in life. Even a person who possesses ten lakhs of rupees may not have even a tenth of the happiness of the beggar who sleeps on the footpath, not if the former does not feel content with his possession, however large it may be.

If you have achieved a sense of contentment in your life you will always concentrate on what you have rather than what you don't and this will ultimately allow you to enjoy eternal happiness, which is already within you.

Who then, will have contentment in life? I have seen many businessmen arguing that if they were to rest content with what they had, how could they earn more? Unfortunately, this mode of thought is regrettable because true success in human life lies not merely in earning money but more in achieving peace of mind.

In other words, contentment can be obtained more easily if you inculcate a spirit of service and sacrifice and come to realize that the pleasure of things is not in their possession but in their use for others. Unless man serves others instead of enjoying things for himself, he will not know how much happiness he can obtain in the process.

For example, say you are very hungry and have two chapatis on your plate; suppose that just then, a hungry dog comes along and you give him one chapati and you make do with one. Just see the happiness and satisfaction you derive and actually feel even though you have not had your fill. How much happiness you will enjoy, eternal happiness. To achieve contentment in life, one must develop the habit of giving, enjoying what you have with others and seeing others happy.

This habit of serving, sacrificing and sharing what you have with others can be only obtained if you have a sense of detachment. Detachment of worldly materials is a very fundamental need for service to others. One must know that when he was born in this world, everything was there and after his death too he will have to leave everything behind and go. You have not brought anything with you when you were born and you will not carry a single tiny thing when you leave this world. In short, you should have a sense of detachment from worldly life. Bear in mind, nothing is yours.

You are the 'NIMIT', instrument of God, and remember always that even one leaf cannot move if His Will is not present. Finally, His Will will be done. You should have the sense of realization that you are separated from the Creator of this world and that your aim should be to reach Him. You have to perform each and every activity with sincerity and with your full ability, with an awareness that you are doing so according to His Will and with a sense of detachment.

If you have detachment or have at least a spirit of detachment, you will have a serving and sacrificing nature, which will give you in turn, contentment of life. Once you have achieved contentment in your life, simplicity will be at your disposal and finally, you will enjoy the fruit of eternal happiness for which you were struggling and starving and which you were trying to obtain in material things, when in fact, they were within you.

The Almighty's blessings will always be with us if we have a sense of detachment, service to others, contentment and simplicity in our lives.

HARI OM TAT SAT

Kishore V Sonpal in 1966

CREATION

Creation is neither good nor bad. It is as it is. It is the human mind that puts all sorts of constructions on it, as we see creation from our own angles and only in ways that suits our own interests.

A woman is just a woman, but one mind calls her 'mother', another calls her 'Sister' and yet another calls her 'aunt' and so on. Men love women, hate snakes and are indifferent to the grass and stone by the roadside. These connections are the cause of all the misery in the world.

Creation is like the Peepal tree, where birds come to eat its fruit or to give shelter to themselves. Even men rest under the tree to cool themselves and take rest. Yet, some men may even hang themselves on the same tree. Yet the tree lives its quiet life, unconcerned with and unaware of the vague uses that it is put to. It is the human mind that is the originator of all the trouble, which then cries for help.

Is God so partial so as to give peace to one and sorrow to another?

In creation, there is room for everything, but men refuse to see the healthy, the good and the beautiful and go on whining like the hungry man who sits beside a plateful of tasty food but instead of stretching out his hand and reaching for the plate to satiate his hunger, prefers to lament. Whose fault lies here? God or Man?

But fortunately for man, God in his infinite mercy, never forsakes him. He always gives him new chances by providing him with Gurus and scriptures to guide him to find the error in his ways and ultimately, to find eternal happiness.

ARCHITECT OF LIFE

You don't try to architect the perfect future. Whether in personal or professional life, you don't call the shots too far. What you do is this: you go down a path every day and look around and ask yourself how you can do better and what twists and turns you need to take. If you need to take a turn, then take it without any hesitation, and then, don't look back. It's about successfully making the right decision every single time rather than having some grand strategy.

LOVE

Love is a quality of the heart and hence, by its very nature, universal and indivisible. Exclusive love for one's family is but a pale shadow of the love that is born of attachment and a sense of possessiveness and is therefore harmful to all concerned. Only he can love all his kith and kin whose heart is large and warm enough to love all human beings.

There is no man in this world who has not had his own ups and downs. Do not be pessimistic. You can make your life happy by changing your angle of vision towards it. It is by cheerfulness that you conquer the darkening influence that seeks to make you feel miserable. Relying on and submitting to God will bring cheer and peace to your heart. You should give up your impatience and worry.

EVERY DAY: A PRAYER

Every day before us, life perishes,
youthfulness wears away.
Days that are gone never return again.
Time is the eater of the universe.
Wealth is as impermanent as a series
of waves in the water.
Life is fleeting like the Lightning.
Therefore, O Lord, save me who has sought refuge at
your feet, right now, with your unbounded grace.

13 INVISIBLE ACTS OF POWER

1. **Hold** open a door.
2. **Smile.**
3. **Offer** a kind word of encouragement.
4. **Give** a compliment.
5. **Listen** without interruption.
6. **Make** a call when your intuition tells you to!
7. **Offer** a prayer for a homeless person.
8. **Pray**–period!
9. **Forgive** others and yourself.
10. **Prepare** a meal for a friend.
11. **Refrain** from judging another person harshly.
12. **Remember** that life is full of miracles and have faith that every difficult situation can change within a blink of the eye.
13. **Remember** the truth that there is no such thing as a small and insignificant act of service.

TEN RULES OF HAPPINESS

1. **Live a simple life**, be temperate in your habits. Avoid self-seeking and selfishness. Make simplicity the keynote of your daily plans. Simple things are the best
2. **Spend less than you earn**. This might be tough in the beginning, but it pays a huge dividend later. Stay out of debt. Cultivate frugality, prudence and self-denial. Avoid extravagance.
3. **Think constructively**. Train yourself to think clearly and accurately. Store your mind with useful thoughts.
4. **Cultivate a yielding disposition.** Resist the common tendency to want things to go your own way. Try to see the other person's point of view.
5. **Be grateful**. Begin the day with an act of gratitude for your opportunities and blessings. Be glad for the privilege of life and work. Rule your moods. Cultivate a mental attitude towards peace and good-will.
6. **Give generously**. There is no greater joy in life than to render joy and happiness to others by means of intelligent giving.
7. **Work with the right motives**. The highest purpose of life should be to grow in spiritual grace and power.
8. **Be interested in others**. Divert your mind from being self-centred. It's the degree to which you give, serve and help others that will determine your level of happiness.
9. Live in a daylight compartment, i.e. **live one day at a time**. Concentrate on the task in hand. Make the most of the day, because that's all you have at the moment.
10. **Have a hobby**; nature walking, gardening, golf, music, photography, etc. Cultivate an avocation to which you can turn to for diversion and relaxation.

CHANGE YOURSELF

'If you hate your present job and long to do something else, then quit your job today.' That is the advice we used to get from counsellors

Then, it was discovered that some do not like their second job any better than the first one. The same is then true for their third job, and so on. The root cause of the problem was not just that they did not like the work, they just did not like working. Before you change your job, make sure you know what you don't like.

Marriage counsellors say 'The reason why marriage is not a success for some people is that they cannot make a success of anything else either.'

So, whether it is your job, hobby, marriage or something else that is not going well, the first thing that you need to do is *change yourself.*

POWER OF OBSERVATION

To understand means to be conscious of; it does not necessarily mean that one has to act definitively in a certain manner. But one has to be conscious of them, aware of them, to know their content, meaning and significance.

Observation is an art. To learn one has to be observed.

Intelligence is not knowledge. A man who has read a lot has accumulated knowledge, but he is not necessarily intelligent. To be intelligent means to be someone one who has the capacity for insight, to see immediately what is true and to make out what is false as well and deny the same. That requires intelligence, which needs to be cultivated. The act of observation requires discipline.

You cannot learn if you are accumulating. Then you belong to the past; you are a dead human being. You only learn if you are living, moving, running, flowing and that demands your complete attention.

9 WAYS TO CHANGE PEOPLE

1. Begin with praise and honest appreciation.
2. Call attention to people's mistakes indirectly.
3. Talk about your own mistakes before criticizing the other person.
4. Ask questions instead of directly giving orders.
5. Let the other man save face.
6. Praise even the slightest improvement. Be hearty in your approbation and lavish in your praise.
7. Give the other person a fine reputation to live up to.
8. Use encouragement. Make the fault seem easy to correct.
9. Make the other person feel happy about doing the things that you suggest.

TRUTH AND HAPPINESS

Only when thought is free from the sensory values, made by the hand or mind, can there be the realisation of truth.

There is no defined path to truth. You must sail on the uncharted sea to find it. Reality cannot be conveyed to another being. For that which is conveyed, is already known. And what is known is not real.

Happiness lies in the freedom that virtue brings. Virtue is not an end in itself, but it is essential for that freedom only so that reality can come into being.

LAW OF MORAL CAUSATION

An aspect of the cosmic order is that it is universal and indestructible.

In accordance with this law:

- If truth is realised, lasting achievements will follow.
- If non-violence is realised, love will be attracted.
- If sexual waste is controlled, vigour will follow.
- If absolute honesty is realised, it will attract riches.
- If non-possession is realised, self-realisation will be reached.

If this law is enacted with a strong will, man and his environment in this life and in the future will be changed so as to secure 'Sarvodaya', the highest good for all.

—Mahatma Gandhi

LYING

The essence of lying is deception but not simply in words; a lie may be told by silence, by equivocation, by a glance of the eye, by attaching a peculiar significance to a sentence.

All these kinds of lies are worse by many degrees than a lie plainly worded.

LOVE AND RELATIONSHIPS

Relationships become of very little significance when based on mutual gratification. Relationships become very significant when it's based on self-revealing.

Love has no relationship. It is only when the other becomes more important than love that there begins a relationship of pain and pleasure.

When you give yourself utterly and wholly, then there is no mutual gratification. Instead begins a process of self-realisation.

There is no gratification in love.

Such love is a marvellous thing. In it, there is no friction; only a state of complete integration of ecstatic beings. There are moments, such rare happy and joyous moments when there is love and complete communion. Love recedes when the object becomes more important, then a conflict of possession and fear begins and love recedes. The further it recedes, the greater the problem of the relationship becomes, losing its meaning. *Love is a state of being when the activities of the self have ceased.*

The present is the only door through which understanding can come into being.

REFUSAL WITHOUT REBUFF

So many foolish people say 'yes' only because they are afraid to refuse a request. And then they spend anxious days finding excuses to break their promise.

When you are afraid to refuse, ask for time to decide. And when you have to refuse, do so with tact and grace, but always with firmness about the decision.

Avoid being rude or crude in your refusal. If you cannot trust yourself with a dominating person, send your refusal in writing.

Tactful people can refuse in such a way to make you feel that you are receiving a favour rather than a snub. Theirs is a refusal without rebuff.

REPENTANCE

A clear confession, combined with a promise to never repeat the sin again, when offered before one who has the right to receive it, is the purest type of repentance.

RECOVERY OF DUES

Do not take any legal action against anybody for recovery of your dues. This step will engender only bitterness, failure and frustration. Impatience denotes lack of trust.

Do not forget the truth that nothing here belongs to you. All, including yourself, belongs to the supreme Lord of the Universe. The sense of possession is one of the main characteristics of the ego sense.

—Swami Ramdas

TRUE LOVE

Love works the most triumphantly in the field of self-suffering and self-sacrifice. It does not seek comfort or gain for itself at the expense of others. Bravely and cheerfully, it endures all pains and sorrows in a spirit of perfect surrender to the will and dispensation of the supreme lord.

Man is miserable because he seeks joy and peace in external conditions and objects, which in their very nature are incapable of yielding the perfect state for which the heart of man longs.

Seek not to transform the world before you have brought the needed change in yourself.

—Swami Ramdas

RISK

If you don't take risks on a new idea, that itself is a risk.

PEACE, MY HEART

Peace, my heart, let the time for the parting be sweet.
Let it not be a death but completeness.
Let love melt into memory and pain into songs.
Let the flight through the sky end in the folding of the wings over the nest.
Let the last touch of your hands be gentle like the flower of the night.
Stand still, O Beautiful End, for a moment, and say your last words in silence.
I bow to you and hold up my lamp to light you on your way.

—Rabindranath Tagore in *The Gardener*, no. 61